# SUPER-CHARGE

## YOUR **STRESS**

## **MANAGEMENT**

## IN THE AGE OF

## **COVID-19**

### A Handbook for Emergency Services and Healthcare Professionals

D1516985

**By Mike Taigman** *and* **Sascha Liebowitz**

Published by Vow3 Publishing
1187 Coast Village Rd. Suite 1
#784
Montecito, CA 93108

9781735049403 (print)
9781735049410 (epub)

Book design and production by Happenstance Type-O-Rama
Typeset in Macklin Tex and Macklin Sans

First Edition

www.combatcovidstress.com

DISCLAIMER

This book is not medical advice or psychotherapy. If you are suffering from symptoms of PTSD, chronic anxiety, or depression, or are thinking about hurting yourself, please put the book down and get proper help from a medical or psychological professional.

# SUPER-CHARGE
### YOUR **STRESS**
# MANAGEMENT
### IN THE AGE OF
# COVID-19

*This book is dedicated to
those who risk their
health and safety taking
care of the rest of us.*

# *Acknowledgments*

As a lifelong student, I've been blessed with hundreds of amazing teachers who have shared their wisdom in classrooms, at workshops, in books and articles, on phone calls, and over shared meals. Most of what's in this book follows the "see one, do one, teach one" guideline used for decades to train surgeons. I'm sharing with you what I've learned from others.

A special thanks to our collaborator Billie Fitzpatrick, who took this book from concept to reality with speed, grace, and humor, generally laughing with us, not at us. Thank you for getting the importance of this subject and giving us the benefit of your great talent. We are also grateful for the creative and thoughtful professionalism of the folks at Happenstance Type-O-Rama, especially Maureen Forys, Rebecca Rider, and Jeff Lytle.

# Contents

# *Introduction*

M y friend Danielle KognizAnce Barnes, an Oakland paramedic, posted this on her Facebook page:

*My oldest daughter kind of broke my heart tonight . . . kids sometimes make you think. Tonight, I was getting my back up uniform together for work tomorrow (we carry a second uniform while on duty), and she asked why I take two and why do I go to work wearing regular clothes, and come home in regular clothes. I simply told her that if I need to change my uniform, like I did today I have an extra one with me and left it at that. Unprompted she looked at me and said, "Momma please don't bring the coronavirus home to us." I about cried, like many others out there my daughters have a parent that works in a busy ER as a nurse and one that works on a busy ambulance as a paramedic.*

I've been honored to work in emergency services for more than 40 years, beginning as a paramedic and now serving public health, hospital, and safety organizations with FirstWatch. My experience has taught me an undeniable truth: the care and safety of patients and communities is directly related to the health and well-being of the frontline professionals who provide care and service to the public.

Since leaving the street, I've spent my career helping emergency management systems develop strategies to better support their frontline folk. The purpose of leadership, in my opinion, is to ensure that frontline professionals have the systems, tools, and resources necessary to do their work effectively. Having been a member of several emergency services leadership teams over the years, I hope the tools in this book will help those of us on the front line as well as those of us whose job it is to support them. We are in this together.

Right now, I'm hearing from friends all over the world who work in paramedic ambulances, hospital emergency departments, intensive care units, patrol cars, on fire rigs, in 911 dispatch centers, combat units, and other critical public service roles. They are all working full-time on reducing the suffering related to COVID-19, and they all describe feeling overwhelmed by the constant stress that comes with caring for patients, serving the public, and serving their communities, while trying, at the same time, to protect their families and themselves.

When I was a street paramedic, I felt honored to know my personal actions were making a direct positive difference in people's lives every day. I also felt personally and saw in my colleagues how the daily stress of showing up and doing what must be done could take a toll, even when there wasn't a major pandemic. I saw firsthand how particularly traumatic calls affected different people in different ways.

After 9/11 there were reports that about 20 percent of people who worked the horrific incident had post-traumatic stress disorder (PTSD) or a post-traumatic stress injury (PTSI). I wondered about the other 80 percent who didn't. What did they have that made them able to go through that intense situation and suffer less than other people?

That inquiry brought me to in-depth studies in psychology, neuroscience, Eastern philosophy, somatic techniques, and mindfulness meditation, which I've been applying personally and teaching to friends and clients in emergency services for years. I have learned from many great teachers and have been honored to be able to share that learning with others in university and professional settings.

Aware that the COVID-19 outbreak was adding an extra layer of non-stop deadly stress to the daily lives of our public health and safety professionals, I wanted to help. I put together a webinar on stress management and had some colleagues send it out to their contacts, hoping a few folks might be interested. In less than five days, 10,600 people registered.

Unfortunately, the webinar system only had the capacity for 3,000, so most had to watch the recording. I've been speaking at conferences for over 40 years and this webinar was my largest audience ever. That gave me a clue more was needed.

We sent an e-mail to the folks who participated in the webinar and asked if they felt better after using any of the techniques I shared. I heard from emergency medicine physicians in New York City, police officers in Ontario, Canada, fire captains, city auditors, veterans with PTSD, prosecutors, probation officers, wildlife officers, EMTs, trauma-focused psychologists, US Air Force fighter pilots, hostage negotiators, teachers, people in the hospital with COVID-19, and hundreds of others. Every single one of them found something they could use to manage their stress, get through a tough shift at work, be present with their kids, or just feel better. The amount of positive feedback from that webinar has been overwhelming.

Most folks on the front line are telling me that they are passionate about what they do; they find purpose and even joy in having to run toward danger rather than away. They also want to continue to do what they do. And yet the personal risks and magnitude of suffering with this pandemic are things no one should have to face alone. And while their jobs are stressful all the time, there is a kind of global uptick in their, and our, collective experience of stress.

My goal with this book is to hopefully help my frontline colleagues, friends, and family not only get through this crisis with less emotional and physical suffering but also use this situation as an opportunity to power-up our stress management techniques. Ultimately, I would like this book to reduce suffering and increase joy, my life goal, which fits perfectly with my employer FirstWatch's stated mission to "Help the Helpers."

The first part of this book explains how stress works in our mind and body. When I give presentations and work with my graduate students, I have learned that most people find it really helpful to know that what they are experiencing is rooted in the design of all human brains, minds, and bodies. I include this science background so that you can better appreciate the suggestions, exercises, and tools, which are all based upon neuroscience, evidence-based research, and peer-reviewed studies. Though some of the practices might feel a little California woo woo, I encourage you to step out of your comfort zone and give a few a try. If something does not fit for you, leave it and move on to something that does. Many folks are surprised to find how easily some of the world's toughest soldiers use some of these techniques, meditate regularly, and discover how and why to share their feelings.

You will find information on how a stress response can be life-saving under the right circumstances, but the wrong kind of stress response going on for too long can cause a host of life-threatening diseases along with depression, anxiety, PTSD, and suicidal thoughts. You'll also see that the stress response is something we can control—we do not need to be victims of our own stress response once we learn how to dial it down and manage it. Awareness of how we personally respond to stress, combined with simple, easy-to-use techniques, gives us a greater ability to not only manage stress, but to use it, so we can work better and live better.

Next, I provide a series of short techniques that you can use right away to dial down stress. These tools don't require special training, a prescription from your physician, or you to admit that you need help—although I suspect that we can all use some help with our stress levels these days.

I recommend that you look for one or two of these techniques that you really want to practice enough so that you can use them without thinking about it in the middle of a tough situation. Mastering a couple will serve you better than trying to remember them all.

The section "Personalize Your Stress Management Toolbox" will help guide you through a quick trial and error process to find which techniques work best for you so that you can get the most out of the time you invest in your personal stress management routine.

Finally, before we get started, I want to point out that I did not write this book alone. My wife Sascha is not only my coauthor but also my wingman, my partner, and my muse. She has touched every page of this book, and though I am the one with the emergency services background, she is the one with writing skills and a deep understanding of how to create a personal wellness routine.

# *Let's Be Real: It's a Battle*

Why should we take time to increase our stress management tools and training right now? Because we have *more* stress. COVID-19 is putting us all in situations, repeatedly and over time, both personally and professionally, that most of us never conceived of before now. We need to increase our internal, personal capacities to effectively meet the greater, external challenges we face with this pandemic so that we can remain centered and grounded, effective at our jobs, and positive about the future. And for this shift to happen, we need to super-charge our stress management strategies.

When you look at the data in recent studies, it's clear that the COVID-19 pandemic is causing significant stress. The frontline healthcare workers in China who were taking care of patients with COVID-19 have shown a 54 percent rate of depression and a 44.6 percent rate of anxiety; 34 percent of them had insomnia and 71.5 percent of them experienced stress and distress.

A March 2020 survey of 3,270 American adults conducted by Elon University found that

* *71.6 percent of them were afraid of a family member developing this illness.*

* *74.4 percent were afraid of losing their job and questioned their ability to make a living at all as a direct result of this pandemic; the same percentage were also worried about its impact on their personal finances, including the decrease in the value of their 401K, their savings, and any stock market investments.*

* *59.3 percent of them were nervous about spreading the virus themselves, particularly since you can be a carrier of the virus without showing the symptoms of being sick.*

* *56.9 percent were afraid of developing the illness themselves.*

* *29.3 percent were afraid of having to go to work while they were sick.*

These results are from a survey of people in the general population, not healthcare and public safety workers, not emergency services providers, paramedics, firefighters, police officers, nurses, and physicians—all of whom we'd expect to have a higher rate of these issues than regular civilians do. Clearly people are anxious about their futures.

My friend Debbie is a police detective in a small Illinois town. Under normal conditions, her daily life is stressful. But now, it's even more so. Her husband, who is undergoing chemotherapy for treatment of prostate and bladder cancer, has suddenly become even more vulnerable to COVID-19 because of his suppressed immune system. Debbie is terrified of catching the virus and bringing it home to her husband.

An emergency medicine physician friend of mine had a young colleague, a previously healthy nurse in her thirties, who was having difficulty breathing while on duty with him. Two weeks later, she collapsed on the job, was intubated, and later died in the intensive care unit from COVID-19.

A paramedic friend of mine who's a single mother with two small kids and no other means of financial support is terrified every time a patient in the back of her ambulance sneezes or coughs—even though she is armored with an N95 mask, goggles, a face shield, bonnet, a gown, and triple gloves, and has the ventilator system in the back of the ambulance turned up full blast. If she becomes sick or dies, she does not know who will take care of her kids.

A critical care physician described having several patients who required ventilators, only to realize that there were not enough to go around. She was forced to make the unimaginably difficult choices about who got the treatment and who didn't.

These are real people whose jobs ask them to go into battle each and every day. And though I've never been to war and don't pretend to know what battle is actually like, when I see friends on the front lines, putting on their face masks, goggles, face shields, gowns, and a triple layer of rubber gloves, I am reminded of the body armor that soldiers, police officers, and some paramedics wear to protect against bullets or fragments of a bomb.

In our case now, the enemy is a microscopic virus that is striking great swaths of people all over the world. And for those who are first responders—in hospitals, ambulances, police cruisers, and fire engines—it's a reality that you could die if your protective gear does not work.

The possibility of losing teammates to injury or death is also real. Anyone working today knows we need to do all we can to stay as strong and healthy as possible—physically and mentally—for ourselves, our families, and the communities we serve. And although it's true that every essential worker will experience some fear, the key is to become aware of how and when we experience fear and channel it effectively.

First, we need to understand that fear is both common and inevitable. We are hard-wired for this emotion to keep us alert to danger or possible threat. Second, we need to allow ourselves to feel fear, accept it, and not try to hide or suppress it. Our fear can protect us and can even save our lives.

## BATTLEMIND

These kinds of issues and life-and-death stressors have led some people to describe the COVID-19 situation we're in as if it were a battle or a war. Some of my friends who've served in the military are uncomfortable with this comparison. Others feel it's an absolutely accurate analogy. As part of my research for this book, I explored the way the US Military, the Army in particular, prepares soldiers emotionally and psychologically for going into battle and managing their stress during battle so that when their service is complete, they retain the highest level of mental and emotional health possible.

I apologize to anyone who has served who might take offense to the notion that the stress associated with battling COVID-19 as a frontline worker is similar to the stress of combat that involves IEDs, tanks, rockets, bombs, and snipers. My intent is not to belittle in any way, shape, or form the service of combat personnel, but to help our frontline people benefit from an incredibly useful framework developed to help those who need to function at the highest levels while under threat of deadly peril.

Specifically, I think that our civilian nurses, physicians, paramedics, firefighters, and police officers can benefit from the concept of *Battlemind*, which was developed by scientists at Walter Reed Army Institute of Research to help prepare soldiers for battle. Battlemind helps focus soldiers on the fact that combat is intense, is potentially life-threatening, and requires a combination of both calm and alertness—the same kind of super-stress management that people working on the front lines of the COVID-19 pandemic or any other crisis situation require to do their best.

## EXPLICIT AND IMPLICIT MEMORY

If you've ever done a squat or push-up or any kind of physical exercise to keep in shape and prevent physical injury, then you get the concept of strengthening for prevention. Those of us who've been bodily injured also have gotten to experience physical therapy for recovery. Like biceps and quads, the brain is a muscle that can be exercised for better injury prevention and optimal functioning even under a high degree of relentless stress.

And just as it's easier to stay in shape than it is to get back in shape once we've been hurt, it's easier to strengthen the brain than it is to wait until we are sidelined, get injured, or develop PTSD. The time is now. It's much more difficult to come back from a trauma than it is to train and strengthen our stress management techniques now. This kind of training also becomes the backbone of our resilience and will help us recover better when or if that becomes necessary.

Building our stress management fitness is similar to sports training, where we train our muscles and practice drills to better our performance and avoid injury. In addition to training to avoid injury when we are doing CPR or disarming an assailant, we can also train our brains to operate most effectively to protect us from stress injuries as we do our jobs during this crisis. That optimal state we are trying to achieve is one where we feel centered and grounded, calm yet alert, confident and energized. We know what to do; we feel prepared and agile; and we move efficiently, as if on automatic. This is what super-stress management is all about.

Just like for any type of training, different people need different amounts of stress management training; everyone starts in a different place, and no matter where we start, how emotionally strong or weak we feel we are right now, making any effort to improve will net rewards for us professionally and personally.

What we want is to get our stress management program into our implicit memory so we can access it without any effort when we need it. In neuroscience, we talk about two different kinds of memory, explicit memory and implicit memory. Think back to when you learned to drive a car. For me, it was the neighbor lady across the street who taught me because my parents were too nervous to be in a vehicle with me. When I was learning to drive, my neighbor took me to an abandoned parking lot and showed me how to use the stick shift and clutch in her 1967ish Ford Mustang—which obviously says something about my age. Pulling that memory out of my past, like pulling a card from a deck in my mind, is explicit memory.

When I get in my car today, I just start it up and drive. I don't have to think about how to use the accelerator, brake, steering wheel, and turn signals. Even though I once learned these steps so that I could drive, I don't need to think about these lessons from the past; I just drive. That's implicit memory. Being able to drive a car, tie your shoes, ride a bike, brush your teeth, or send a text are all examples of implicit memory in action.

It's well worth the time investment to have at least one stress management technique that becomes part of your implicit memory so that when you're in the middle of an intensely stressful situation, you can dial down your stress automatically without having to "remember" a technique consciously.

And this is what we aim for when we learn techniques for more effective stress management. When we are working long, hard hours, and we are on the front lines of whatever job we're in, we can use one or more of these strategies to stay calm and focused during a prolonged crisis. When we're in the middle of working in a dangerous area, which could be any place in the world at this point in time, and we have to recall our stress management techniques with explicit memory in order to activate them, they'll be less helpful to us than if we train to make them implicit memory. Imagine if every time a bug flew in our eye we had to think "blink." We would have had several preventable eye injuries by now.

On the other hand, if we put in the practice and make some go-to techniques so familiar that they become part of implicit memory, then there's a much better chance we will use them when the time comes, and be better at doing so.

Most of the techniques in this book take less than 2 minutes to try. Some will make more sense than others. Some will feel more natural, like extensions of strategies you are already using. Some of these tips might require more time to learn or get used to. But know this: all of them will help, because they all train the brain to stay calm, focused, and energized while working this high-intensity crisis.

One of the first stress management lectures I ever attended was given by a physician during a continuing education session at St. Joseph's Hospital in Denver, Colorado. It was 1980 and the doctor said, "When you're faced with stress, you can do one of three things. You can get away from it, you can try to change the source of it, or you can change your own perspective/reaction to it."

The COVID-19 virus is not something we can get away from or change today. It's here, it's worldwide, and it's not going away any time soon. We have hope for better tests, vaccines, and treatments, but as of this writing, these are not options at our fingertips.

Therefore, our only option is to reduce the stress associated with COVID-19 and change our perspectives and reactions from the inside out. Once we put our reactions to the pandemic squarely in the category of things *inside* our control, we can say to ourselves, "Yes, I have anger, sadness, and fear toward the situation, but these emotions will not help me get through each day better."

Then it's time to get real and learn how to dial down those feelings and get to that centered, calm, focused, energized state, *despite* our feelings. Cultivating that centered, powerful way of being will help all of us get through this together and save lives, maybe even some of our own.

And there's good news. We can learn to control how we respond to stress. Thanks to the science of learning and neuroplasticity, we can train our brains, minds, and bodies to respond more effectively to both chronic and acute stress, the stress of this pandemic, and other sources of preexisting stress that we have. Decreasing the negative impacts of stress on our body, mind, and performance at work are key aspects of the brain/mind stress management training techniques offered in this book. I hope these exercises and techniques also offer you an extra boost to make you feel even more confident handling your own anxiety, fatigue, and other effects of non-stop stress.

Another benefit of learning these techniques is that we can share them with our friends, colleagues, and families. We can up our leadership skills by prioritizing mental and emotional strength training, knowing that we are helping others.

Just as we can have some influence on the physical health of our communities by encouraging people to follow the practices that decrease the spread of the virus or the likelihood that they transmit it or get sick themselves, we can help others by guiding them to focus on what they can change in themselves to feel better during this time rather than on what they can't change out in the world.

The choice is clear. Changing our perspective and our reaction to the stresses caused by this pandemic is the option that puts us more in control and has the best likelihood of success.

# *A Personal Story of Crisis Rehearsal*

E arly in my career, when I was working as a street paramedic, I was on Ambulance 4 one evening. We had just dropped a patient off at Denver General Hospital when we got a call to 40 South Pennsylvania for an officer down.

A woman had called 911 because she was afraid her drunk husband might kill her. The patrol car dispatched to the house contained a field training officer and a rookie officer halfway through his training in the Denver Police Academy.

When the officers pulled up near the front of the house, they noticed a man standing behind the screen door with a long-barrel firearm and called in the situation as a man with a gun. Shortly after that, the man inside the house started firing at the patrol car.

The field training officer took a position of cover behind a parked car across the street and the rookie officer took up a position of cover behind a four-foot-high concrete retaining wall in front of the guy's house, which was up on a little bit of a hill. As they were shooting back and forth, the rookie officer looked up to return fire and took a shotgun blast to the forehead, which dropped him on the sidewalk.

That's when the field training officer called in officer down. We responded and took up a position of cover a half block away behind a large apartment complex. Because it was nighttime, when my partner and I did a quick look around the side of the apartment complex, we could see flashes of gunfire going back and forth between the man with the long-barrel firearm, the field training officer, and several other officers who had arrived on scene.

Somebody on the police radio suggested that the lights in the neighboring houses were back-lighting officers approaching, making them targets. Almost immediately, all the officers on the scene shot out all of the streetlights and all of the front porch lights on the houses up and down the street with a shower of gunfire and broken glass.

My partner and I were now in almost pitch black. As I peeked out again, I saw a friend of mine, a sergeant, who was trying to approach the downed officer, get shot in the chest. He dropped to the ground next to the first downed officer. So now we had two downed officers in the middle of an ongoing gunfight in the dark.

The Denver SWAT team arrived behind the apartment complex, as well as a pumper from the Denver Fire Department. We quickly hatched a plan to put one of the SWAT team's ballistic shields in the window of the pumper on the gunman's side. Then my partner, two EMTs from the Denver Fire Department, the SWAT officers, and I would ride on the far side of the pumper as it drove to the injured. So now we were riding on the running board on the far side of a fire truck driving down the street into the firefight.

The SWAT team told us they were going to fire 30 seconds' worth of nonstop gunfire into the house to give us time to extract the downed officers and bring them behind the safety of the pumper.

As they started the firing, we extricated the officers and backed the pumper down the street to where another paramedic ambulance had joined. We put one officer into each ambulance, and took them both to Denver General Hospital.

The rookie succumbed to his injuries and my sergeant friend went into cardiac arrest. When we moved him over to the bed in the trauma center at Denver General, they opened up his chest. They were successfully able to patch and restart his heart. He survived, was discharged, and went back to work the streets in Denver until his retirement.

Although this was one of the most stressful situations I have ever experienced, when I think of it now, I believe that all the crisis rehearsal I had done for worst-case scenarios before that moment allowed me to keep a cool head and function effectively so that I could lead my team through that extrication process. That training also probably saved the life of my friend in the process.

## REHEARSE THE CRISIS TECHNIQUE

In the late 1980s, I was introduced to the concept of *crisis rehearsal*, a mental practice and preparation technique, during a law enforcement Street Survival Seminar put on by Calibre Press. Calibre was, at that time, the number one educator for police officers on street survival and defensive tactics.

In the training, they taught us to imagine a crisis situation of some kind and imagine it vividly. The trainers asked us to imagine the sights, the smells, and the sounds of a particular scenario. One scenario that I used to practice imagining frequently when I was working as a street paramedic was being confronted with an angry person with a firearm. I would imagine those situations vividly and think through strategies of how I could get myself, my partner, and our patient through them alive.

Once we brought a scene to life in our heads, the trainers told us to think through different strategies to get out of the situation successfully. Like in sports, we always want to practice winning, survival, and success. Like athletes, we also do drills to strengthen our skills, reaction times, and other parts of the sport, game, or in our case, crisis situation.

According to author, medical school professor, and clinical psychiatrist Dan Siegel, "Neurons that fire together wire together." When we practice imagining ourselves getting through difficult situations successfully, we are wiring our brains to anticipate success and automatically look for ways to be successful any time we're faced with a challenge. When the brain anticipates success and stays in a frame of mind where success feels likely, it is better positioned, chemically and neurologically, to be successful.

This does not mean we can "think ourselves" into *not* contracting COVID-19, but we can rehearse taking the actions we need to take to stay healthy ourselves while taking care of others. The crisis

---

## TRY IT: REHEARSE A CRISIS

1. Bring to mind a possible crisis scenario.

2. Imagine your actions from beginning to end, step by step.

3. Fill in the imagined scenario with details such as smells, sounds, and visuals that help to bring the scenario to life.

4. Now visualize the successful outcome to that event.

Any time you want to practice crisis rehearsal, go through a similar sequence of imagined actions and reactions. This kind of worst-case scenario preparation will help you when the time comes.

---

rehearsal technique improves the chances that when life throws you a real situation similar to the one you've rehearsed, you'll feel better able to handle it, staying centered, grounded, and efficient with your energy and your focus. This attitude and state of mind will help you succeed.

# *Understand Your Stress Response*

Why is it so hard sometimes for us to stay calm during stressful situations even when we're telling ourselves, "Stay calm"? It's like we know what we're supposed to do, but sometimes a stronger force takes over. To prep for how to boost our stress management, let's walk through a bit about how stress works in our brains.

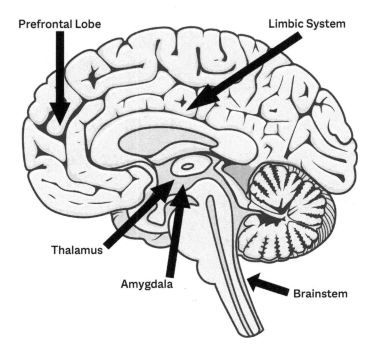

Prefrontal Lobe

Limbic System

Thalamus

Amygdala

Brainstem

As you can see from the diagram, the brainstem is the base of our brain. It essentially differentiates us from a head of cabbage and makes sure we breathe. It also regulates other basic functions, including swallowing, blood pressure, heart rate, and temperature.

The next part of the brain is our limbic system, which is where our most primal emotions are generated. Love, joy, and happiness, along with fear, anger, and depression, live in our limbic system.

The neocortex or prefrontal cortex (PFC), the outer edge of our brain, is the thinking part. When it comes to dealing with stress, we use the PFC to make conscious decisions, including how to *strategize* when we are confronted with a challenge or crisis. The PFC is in charge of so-called higher-order reasoning, executive decision-making, and impulse control. Whatever you're thinking about right now as you're reading this sentence is happening in the PFC. When we're cut off in traffic and our first thought is to honk loudly on the horn and wave at the other driver with just one finger, it's the executive center, that helps exercise control over this impulsive response and gives us the power to make choices that are less likely to get us shot by the other driver.

## YOUR BRAIN'S ANATOMY

It can be helpful to have a basic understanding of how the brain works so that you can better appreciate how the stress management techniques work. Neuroscience is pretty complicated but here's a super-simple cheat sheet:

**Brainstem**—The base of the brain that controls basic body functions like breathing and body temp regulation.

**Limbic System**—The seat of all our emotions.

**Prefrontal Lobe**—Also known as the "thinking brain," or the "executive center." It's where conscious thinking happens.

**Thalamus**—The brain's communications center. It takes information from all the senses and sends it to other parts of the brain for analysis and possible action.

**Amygdala**—The body's lifeguard and alarm system.

**Nervous System**—All of the brain and its functions are part of the nervous system, along with the spinal cord, sensory organs, and nerves.

**Parasympathetic Response**—The relaxation response, which includes feelings of love and happiness.

**Sympathetic Response**—The stress response, which includes feelings of fear or excitement.

It's worth noting that when we consume alcohol, we lose some of this impulse control; the prefrontal cortex is sedated, which is why people sometimes do things they later regret as a result of alcohol intoxication.

The next part of the brain is the thalamus, which essentially works as the communication center. Like a 911 dispatch center, it takes in information from the optic nerve, the auditory nerve, proprioception, and other senses and routes this information to the appropriate other parts of the brain for analysis and potential action.

Sitting on either side of the thalamus are two little pieces of neurologic tissue called the amygdala. These little almond-shaped pieces are key to understanding how stress works in ourselves, our work colleagues, and our friends or family members. I first learned about the amygdala (a part of the limbic system) from Daniel Goleman and his book *Emotional Intelligence*. The amygdala essentially serves as our body's lifeguard. It's on duty 24 hours a day, 7 days a week, 365 days a year, and it evaluates every sight, smell, and sound that we run across in our lives.

The amygdala asks three questions of everything that it perceives:

1. *"Is this something I can mate with?"*

2. *"Is this something I can eat?"*

3. *"Is this something that is likely to eat me?" (something life-threatening)*

If it gets a "no" answer to these questions, it essentially does nothing. On the other hand, if it gets a "yes," it activates a cascade of neurochemicals that inspire emotions, feelings.

If the answer to the question "Can I mate with it?" is "yes," it activates the systems that cause the emotions of joy, happiness, or love—in other words, a relaxation response.

On the other hand, if the answer to the question "Is this something that's going to eat me?" is "yes," then it activates either a flight, fight, freeze, or faint response.

Most of us learned the flight or fight response back in biology class, but since then, I've learned from Dan Siegel that some people freeze and others faint. A theory that's been floated is that this biologic response is related to why some animals faint and pretend they are dead—so they won't be eaten by predators who like their meal to be alive and kicking. These responses are all part of our built-in survival mechanisms that protect us from danger and threats.

But these automatic stress responses can impair our thinking brain's ability to control our thoughts, emotions, and actions. Most of us, most of the time, do want our thinking brain in the driver's seat, which is why learning techniques to dial down the stress response is so important, especially for people who work in emergency services or healthcare.

Because the connection between the amygdala and the thalamus is a fairly thin pathway, the amygdala has to make a very quick assessment as to whether or not something poses a danger based on a vague impression of what's happened out there. For this reason, it has the potential to ring the alarm bells when situations are *not* really a threat. Have you ever jumped at the sound of a slamming door? Or cried out when you were surprised? This is your amygdala overreacting: the loud or surprising noise triggers a threat response even though it's not warranted.

Another important feature of our limbic system is that its wiring and degree of sensitivity vary a lot from person to person. Sensitivity can also change in the same person at different times, depending on other factors in their lives such as how much sleep they had the night before, whether they are having relationship issues that day, or if they've just come from dealing with another highly stressful situation.

Some of us can remain cool as cucumbers even when we are facing a situation that might be terrifying for others. Others of us—because of our particular genetic makeup and lived experience—may have more sensitive or reactive wiring.

Here's an example from the movie *Free Solo*, in which the free climber Alex Honnold climbs some of the world's highest and most difficult cliffs without ropes or protection. When I saw the film, I gripped the sides of the theater seat for fear I was going to fall as Alex climbed 7,569-foot El Capitan in Yosemite Valley with no ropes or protection of any kind. And yet was Alex scared while he actually did the climbing?

No. Well, at least not biologically. When they did a functional magnetic resonance imaging (fMRI) scan of Alex's brain, they found that situations that frighten most of us don't activate his amygdala at all.

## PARASYMPATHETIC AND SYMPATHETIC NERVOUS SYSTEM

The autonomic nervous system comprises both the sympathetic nervous system and the parasympathetic nervous system. The sympathetic nervous system prepares the body for intense physical activity, usually in response to a threat or a challenge. It increases heart rate, tenses the muscles, and improves alertness.

The parasympathetic nervous system does the opposite. It relaxes the body and inspires a state of calm. The heart rate slows and the muscles relax. When we strive for that centered, grounded-yet-alert state for dealing with high stress situations, we want these two systems to be in balance. The techniques in this book are designed to do just that.

We each have our own level of reactivity. Some people have a hair-trigger stress response and some people take a while to respond, but we all have a response system.

The stress response system evolved way back when we were foraging for our food and living in caves; it's part of our built-in survival mechanism. Those of us who work in emergency services need to understand and rely on this part of our nervous system.

If you're a first responder taking care of a situation in the living room in somebody's house on a 911 call and you hear the sound of a shotgun being racked in the next room along with an angry voice, you will automatically and immediately back out of the room. If you're a law enforcement officer, you may draw your own weapon to try to deal with the threat.

Most mammals are equipped with a version of this system. The difference between humans compared to the rest of the animal world is that we have this big brain that has the ability to imagine threats that trip our stress response. We worry and create loops in our heads that constantly activate our stress response. It's these loops, or patterns, that can cause many of the problems associated with long-term stress, or PTSD.

The consequences of unmanaged chronic stress are many and varied. Have you heard of vicarious trauma? Critical incident stress? Secondary trauma? Compassion fatigue? Burnout? These names of conditions are all kind of the same wine in a different bottle; they are all manifestations of unmanaged stress.

There are a number of physiologic consequences to prolonged stress. At the level of our body's cells, the *mitochondria*, the little battery packs inside our cells that generate energy, can become damaged and less functional. Inflammation is another part of the stress response and the body's immune response. One type of inflammation is the immediate swelling that happens after an injury or laceration, or the blisters we get when we burn ourselves that launch the healing process. However, when the body gets stuck in a cycle of chronic inflammation—from dealing ineffectively with an ongoing crisis—then all sorts of bad things can occur. Free radicals attack and damage cells through oxidative stress, which decreases their functioning and ultimately undermines the immune system. This chronic inflammation is also a setup for cardiovascular disease, neurologic disease, autoimmune diseases like rheumatoid arthritis and lupus, fibromyalgia, chronic fatigue, and even cancer.

Each of the strands of DNA in our bodies have caps called *telomeres*. Professor Elissa Epel of University of California, San Francisco (UCSF), explains that telomeres are like the end caps on our shoelaces. They keep the DNA from unraveling. When we are born our telomeres are long, and over the course of our lives they shorten. Some of the things we are exposed to in the world lengthen our telomeres and others shorten them.

Researchers have found that the length of telomeres correlates with a longer life and less disease. They've also seen evidence that exposure to things like chronic emotional or psychological stress, smoking, a diet made up of processed foods, particularly those that are high in added sugar, and a whole pile of other things that your parents probably told you not to do contribute to a shortening of telomeres.

Telomere length—short or long—is ultimately part of aging, which determines how long we live. So it's in our best interest to lengthen our telomeres and lengthen our lives. How? By more effectively reducing and managing our stress. Eating fruits, vegetables, and whole grains; getting deep and restful sleep; spending time in nature; and practicing mindfulness can all help us increase and lengthen our telomeres.

Stress-related oxidation, inflammation, and shortened telomeres contribute to all kinds of health problems including high blood pressure, obesity, diabetes, cardiovascular disease, neurovascular disease, all types of cancer, and any of the more than 100 autoimmune diseases.

Chronic unmanaged stress has emotional and psychological impacts on us as well. It is associated with depression, anxiety, burnout, and compassion fatigue. It is a setup to acquire PTSD and can even lead some people to suicidal thoughts or actions.

But remember: stress is necessary for us to survive. It keeps us alive during times when we need it to kick in and tell us to freeze, flee, fight, or faint. It's absolutely crucial during a combat situation and when you're an essential worker, helping your community during a viral pandemic.

Stress keeps us vigilant and ready to respond to dangers. It keeps us paying attention to our personal protective equipment (PPE) even when it's uncomfortable, or when the goggles fog up. Stress

## CHECK IN: HOW SENSITIVE IS YOUR STRESS RESPONSE?

Do you notice that you're more easily startled than other folks, or do you tend to be the calm one in a group?

Do you spend more time helping others calm down or are folks more likely to spend time talking you down?

This self-assessment of your own system can help make you more aware of your current default way of reacting so you know what you're working with. If your system seems overreactive or if you startle easily, you may want to try some relaxation techniques (see pages 38-39). If you tend to be less reactive, you may want to practice crisis rehearsal (see page 18) to make sure you feel prepared to act decisively during a crisis.

helps keep you focused, even when that mask just gets nasty and you feel like it's awful to have to reuse something that you used to use just one time and throw out. Being vigilant can also help protect us against COVID-19 and help us protect those we love and care about. And being able to do that is important.

There's an edge we need to walk: we need a healthy stress response to alert us so that we maintain safety practices and avoid dangerous situations. But we also need to learn to manage the impacts of prolonged or intense stress effectively so we can mitigate the negative side effects such as PTSD, heart disease, and other potential physical or psychological conditions.

# STRESS

# MANAGEMENT

# **TECHNIQUES**

# First, Calm Your Body

A basic step in super-charging your stress management is learning easy ways to calm your body—you consciously direct your body to relax and, as a result, reduce anxiety. Eating well, exercising, getting enough rest, and staying away from toxins like alcohol, drugs, and tobacco also help your body stay calm.

## EAT, MOVE, SLEEP

A first step in building a strong stress response is making sure that you eat well, move a little, and sleep well. When we treat our body with care, we help regulate our parasympathetic nervous system, which helps us relax, and we support our immune system, both of which play an important role in how we manage stress.

## Eat

One of my go-to sources for reliable nutrition information is Dr. Dean Ornish, who pioneered a lot of the research that established lifestyle medicine. He recently published a book with his wife Anne Ornish called *UnDo It!*, which describes the Ornish lifestyle program, which is now covered by Medicare because it so clearly prevents and reverses many chronic diseases.

Dr. Ornish's approach to health is quite simple: eat well, move more, stress less, and love more. This framework has been shown to dramatically improve health and longevity. The guidelines and recipes are really clear. Eating more plants, less processed foods, and less added sugar is the recipe for a healthier, less stressful life.

One of the challenges of being in a chronically stressful situation is that stress tends to inspire people to seek out sugars, fats, and fast, easy-to-down foods. It seems easier to grab donuts, pizzas, hamburgers, and french fries quickly and shove them in your face when you're in a hurry and you're stressed than take the time to eat a salad or make a lentil soup or eat something that is healthier. But if we can bring ourselves to do it, we'll get benefits from eating fresh fruits, vegetables, and whole grains, and avoiding the processed foods, added sugars, and high fat.

I am in no position to give anybody weight loss or diet advice, but I encourage all who are curious to read Dean and Anne Ornish's book or either of Dr. Michael McGregor's books, *How Not to Die* or *How Not to Diet*. All three books are jam-packed with rock-solid scientific research on nutrition and its relationship to health and longevity, and I really encourage you to check them out.

One thing about unhealthy eating is it can be a way to feel good momentarily, but it sets us back in the long run. Substituting an apple or two for a donut once in a while can make a difference. Choosing trail mix instead of chips or water instead of soda are body/mind-positive choices that can have an impact on our ability to manage stress effectively.

## Move

So how do we fit in movement? When we're exhausted, it's hard to find the extra time to exercise, but adding even 15 or 20 minutes of movement to our day makes a huge difference. Try parking a long way from where you need to go to get a good walk in or taking the stairs instead of the elevator (of course, be careful not to touch the bannisters!)—these are easy ways to make your body move.

We can re-create triathlons or build a CrossFit gym in our living room if we're so inspired, but we don't need to. Neuroscience researcher Bruce Perry says, "Just 90 seconds of movement is enough to re-regulate our nervous system."

Even the most sedentary of us can march in place, do 10 squats, flow through a single yoga sun salutation (Google it!), or dance to our favorite tune for 90 seconds. And it's worth it. Short frequent doses of movement throughout the day increase our endurance and improve our performance while decreasing our stress response. One way to help remember to pack movement into our day is to pair it with another regular daily activity, like marching in place while we brush our teeth, doing lunges while the coffee is brewing, or enjoying some gentle shoulder and neck rolls when we sit down.

When you have more time for exercise when you're not at work, it's good to find something you enjoy doing while making sure that you're not sharing the virus. There are thousands of workouts to do at home including yoga, body-weight strength builders, and virtual martial arts or dance classes. Use your favorite internet search engine to find something that's fun for you.

## Sleep

I cannot underestimate the importance of sleep. When I first started learning about and really understanding the science of resilience, what caught my attention was the role of sleep in how our body can restore itself. This information hit me right in the face because of my lifelong belief that I only needed four or five hours of sleep a night.

I thought that four or five hours was just plenty. What I soon learned was that my body and brain's lack of sufficient sleep was causing me to be both prediabetic and obese. The lack of sleep also was exacerbating my asthma. Sleep, it turns out, has a major impact not only on metabolism and body regulation but also on brain functioning. The main ingredient that enables the body to restore itself is the quantity and quality of *deep* sleep.

According to the American Academy of Sleep Medicine, "Adults should sleep 7 or more hours per night on a regular basis to promote optimal health." Less than 7 hours a night on a regular basis is associated with adverse health outcomes including obesity, diabetes, high blood pressure, heart disease, stroke, depression, poor performance, and increased risk of death.

So how do we make sure we get enough deep sleep?

One incredibly helpful tool that I use is a wearable. My choice is the Apple Watch because it tracks sleep duration, how much deep sleep I get, my heart rate, and the quality of my sleep. I use the sleep tracker system to make sure I at least stay in bed and give myself the opportunity for 7 to 8 hours of sleep each night. Just resting, without any activity, sound, or other distractions, can be beneficial for the body and brain even if it's not full sleep.

In a personal experiment, I tried to improve the depth and length of my sleep by tracking the feedback my watch gives me every morning. I've never been a big drinker of alcohol but I was curious about what effect it had on my sleep. I found that if I had no alcohol at all, I would get about 7 or so hours of good-quality sleep with around 2 hours of that being deep sleep. After just one beer or glass of wine— so I did not get the feeling of intoxication at all—I only got 4 hours of sleep and zero deep sleep. Yes, I've tried this experiment more than once in the hope that it might have been an anomaly, but I get the same result every time.

I've shared these results with a number of other friends who have tried similar experiments on themselves, and they've discovered, to their surprise, that the nightcap they were enjoying in order to sleep better wrecks their sleep. Those of us motivated to get deep sleep on a regular basis might want to try skipping the bedtime beer or nightcap.

---

## TIPS FOR GETTING BETTER SLEEP

Decrease the use of caffeine. Even those people who say that they can drink two pots of coffee and still fall asleep are probably not getting the quality sleep they might believe they are.

Turn off screens including TVs, computers, tablets, phones, and e-readers at least 30 to 60 minutes before bedtime. Try switching to reading a non-work-related book, the kind with actual paper pages, before bed.

Those of us who are nappers need to keep naps to 20 minutes or less and take them more than 6 hours before bedtime. I love naps on the rare day when I can get them. If I take one that's longer than 30 minutes, though, it's a guarantee that I won't sleep well that night. Nappers who are having trouble sleeping when it's bedtime might want to experiment with cutting out naps for a week to see if that helps.

Using the structured worry/stimulus control training technique (see pages 61–62) outlined in this book more than 3 hours before bedtime can help with falling asleep. Also, a cool room temperature with a warm bed and no light is the ideal environment for good sleep.

---

Alcohol, like sugary, salty, or fatty food that seems like a good way to feel better in the moment, actually undermines our immune system and lowers our ability to manage stress over time.

## JUST BREATHE: TACTICAL BREATHING

It often strikes people as a little bit funny to talk about breathing as a stress management technique—after all, we have to breathe all day, every day. In addition to keeping our bodies filled with oxygen and cleared of carbon dioxide, certain breathing patterns can be powerful stress reducers.

In this section, let's focus on what's referred to as *tactical breathing*, also known as *box breathing*. It was made popular by military and law enforcement trainer Lieutenant Colonel Dave Grossman with his book *On Combat*.

Grossman looks at what happens to the human body under the stresses of battle, and the impact of this stress on the nervous system, heart, breathing, auditory perception, and memory—many of the physiological aspects of stress that we've been talking about so far. He describes tactical breathing as a strategy to employ to keep us in the fight and help us survive.

. . . . . .

### *"I've been through critical incidents, and deep breathing works really well."*

—DEPUTY CHIEF JOHN SHORT,
Monterey Bay Police Department

. . . . . .

This breathing technique has been used successfully by the US Military for a long time. Many professional and college athletes also use tactical breathing to gain control of their emotions and manage their stress to achieve optimal performance. Such breathing techniques can also be utilized by frontline professionals.

There are a lot of different ways to make tactical breathing complex, but I find it's best to keep it super simple. This is how it works:

1. *Inhale to a count of four.*

2. *Hold your breath for a count of four.*

3. *Exhale or blow out for a count of four.*

4. *Hold your breath again for a count of four.*

5. *Repeat three or four times.*

Some people find it helpful to visualize a box like the one in this picture. You can try it right now. Inhale 1, 2, 3, 4. Hold 1, 2, 3, 4. Exhale 1, 2, 3, 4. Hold 1, 2, 3, 4. Repeat.

Other forms of breath training are included in many contemplative traditions like Buddhist and Jewish Kabbalistic meditation. It's a regular part of many yoga practices. Breath work is also the

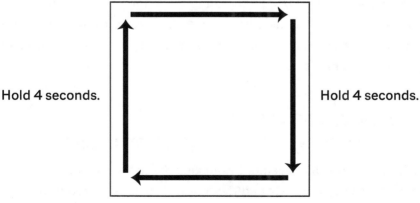

**Breathe in 4 seconds.**

**Hold 4 seconds.**            **Hold 4 seconds.**

**Breathe out 4 seconds.**

foundation for some approaches to psychotherapy like Holotropic Breathwork created by psychiatrist Stanislav Grof.

Another version of breathwork that can calm your body was designed to be more meditative and less tactical. It comes from the Vietnamese Buddhist teacher Thich Nhat Hanh. I was first introduced to this technique during a retreat he led in Northern California. I remember him saying something like this:

> *When you take a breath in, take it in through your nose and visualize the breath coming up over the top of the inside of your head, and cascading calmly all the way down your spine to the bottom of your spinal cord. Then exhale through your mouth slowly, and just as you get toward the end of your exhale, allow your lips to come into a smile, a gentle, natural smile.*

I'm not sure why, but for me, that little smile at the end of a slow, deep, relaxing breath has a really powerful, instantaneous, stress-reducing impact on my body. These breathing patterns can be done anywhere at any time to relax our body, clear our mind, and let our parasympathetic nervous system do its job to help us relax.

In these practices, or any time we bring attention to our breath and consciously slow our breathing by extending the inhale and exhale, we calm our nervous system. The body calms. The mind calms. Breathwork is a reliable stress reliever for whenever we feel the tension begin to build.

## GENERATE GRACE:
## FIVE POWERFUL RELAXATION TECHNIQUES

Like most stress management strategies, the GRACE techniques calm and focus both the body and the mind. I learned them from the late Aikido instructor George Leonard, who was one of the cofounders of the Esalen Institute, a place where I've studied frequently. Leonard was also the author of several popular books including *Mastery*. He describes GRACE as a powerful strategy for tricking the nervous system into feeling relaxed.

GRACE stands for ground, relax, aware, center, energize. It uses the principles of somatic psychology to use the body to reverse the impact of stress by activating the vagus nerve to turn on our parasympathetic response and keep our body/mind calm.

One of the best ways for us to practice the five components of GRACE is to start by standing and bringing our body into a state of extreme physical stress: clench the fists, tighten the shoulders, clench the jaw, squeeze the glutes, and take shallow, fast breaths.

Yes, I'm asking you to try this right now while you're reading this book. And yes, you'll feel silly, but there's no better way to learn this technique than to try it. Now, let everything relax, unclench, and untighten. Take a deep, long inhale, and exhale. Now we're ready to practice the GRACE techniques.

## G Is for Grounding

Part of the automatic stress response is decreased sensation in our arms, hands, legs, and feet. It's designed so that if we get bitten by a predator, it doesn't hurt too badly and we're still able to flee or fight. But grounding does the opposite in that it brings awareness to our toes, which activates the relaxation response.

To practice this grounding strategy:

1. *First, bring awareness to your toes.*

2. *Next, reach out through your toes, imagining that you are trying to grab a carpet or rug and pull it back to bunch up under your toes.*

3. *Next, work your toes like you are trying to get the entire carpet or rug under your feet.*

This action brings your awareness powerfully to your feet, activates the relaxation response, and gives you that sense of having your feet on the ground.

. . . . . .

*"I've tried this technique.*
*I don't know why but*
*it calms me and feels good."*

—CAPTAIN CHRISTOPHER SHERRY,
California Highway Patrol

. . . . . .

## R Is for Relaxing

We all hold our stress differently. I tend to hold it in my neck and shoulders. Other people hold it in their fists. Some people hold it in their bellies. The key for this part of GRACE is to focus on relaxing and moving the one part of your body where you tend to hold stress. For me that means letting my shoulders feel like they are a shirt hanging on a hanger with no effort.

Where in your body do you hold your stress? Take in a deep breath and imagine moving that breath into that part of your body that holds the stress. Next, blow the stress out with your exhale. You can also try wiggling the part around a little bit and just shaking the tension out of just that part of your body.

Without even realizing it, a lot of people also hold tension in their jaw. Try this: let your jaw fall open and let your mouth hang open softly for a second. I know—you may feel a little weird, but try it anyway. Just let your jaw drop open right now. Just ah. More than likely, you will feel a little cascade of relaxation move through your system.

## A Is for Becoming Aware

The A stands for awareness, and in this case, we are becoming aware of our body sensations. When we start to get stressed, most of us experience a tightening or pressure beginning to happen. The key is to notice that sensation; become aware of what happens in the body and where this tension tends to go or affect you.

When we are aware of our body tension, then we can release it rather than going through our day all tensed up physically. Learning to notice and then release tension in the body is what awareness training is about.

Try this quick exercise:

1. *Sitting down, bring to mind a situation that is mildly stressful.*

2. *Next, close your eyes and begin to do a body scan, "visiting" the areas of your body, beginning with your eyes, your ears, and your jaw.*

3. *Do you sense any tension in any of these areas?*

4. *Next, notice your breath. Is it even? Rapid?*

5. *How is the skin on your hands? Tight? Tingly? Moist?*

6. *As you visit all the areas of your body, become aware of any sensations—pleasant or unpleasant. Next, check out your vision, hearing, jaw muscles; notice your breathing—can you feel your heartbeat? What do you notice first?*

Becoming aware of how your body reacts to stress is hugely important because often the body signals the first sign of stress. If we're attuned to our body's sensations, we can catch and manage the reaction before it becomes more intense or takes greater hold. Try to check in with yourself and do quick body scans whenever you notice yourself tightening up. Become aware of whatever your stress signs are. Look for them and say to yourself, "I'm starting to feel stressed." Just noticing and labeling the sensations decreases your stress response.

## C Is for Centering

The fourth step in GRACE is about centering. In martial arts, beginners usually have awkward upper body technique until they learn the concept of physical and emotional centering. If you've ever watched a Steven Seagal movie, you may have noticed how calm and centered he looks as he moves through fight scenes. When we're centered in our bodies, it helps our thoughts become clearer and our actions more deliberate.

Here's how you can connect to your center:

1. *Think about the center of your body as about two inches beneath your belly button.*

2. *Now find that spot on your belly and gently hold your hand on it while at the same time taking a breath in and bringing your attention to that center spot, feeling it expand as you inhale.*

3. *Next, exhale and let your hand move toward your spine as your belly releases and softens.*

4. *Take another deep breath in and try to push your hand out with your breath.*

Going through this belly breathing exercise not only relaxes you, it helps you center yourself—the combination of these effects offers you an extra stress reduction technique.

## E Is for Energize

Energizing is really about warming up the temperature of our hands and feet. Part of the normal stress response is an automatic constriction of the peripheral vessels, making our hands and feet cold. You may have noticed this response when you've touched a friend or partner's hand when they're particularly nervous and realized instantly how cold it was.

We also know how deeply relaxing it feels to get into a warm or hot bath or a hot tub. Heat dilates the blood vessels in our fingers and toes and activates the vagus nerve; this parasympathetic response keeps us calm and centered.

Warming our hands and feet tells our body and mind to relax, and relaxing tells our hands and feet to get warmer. So rubbing hands together to heat them up can help us stay centered and calm. Of course, if you're in a place where you can take a bath or get in a hot tub, go for it.

Each of the GRACE techniques can be done in the moment while at work or at home. Most people find one or two favorites and focus on using the ones they like best. As with all of these tools and techniques, the best one is the one you'll use.

So maybe it's wiggle-the-toes day and that's all it takes, every once in a while, to trigger a relaxation response that helps keep you calm, focused, and energized throughout the day. Doing just that, regularly, can help train the mind to come back to that place of centeredness despite what is going on around you.

# Use the Power of Your Brain

Directing our thoughts is a powerful strategy for reducing anxiety, shifting our perspective, and tapping into our confidence and skills to manage a crisis effectively and successfully. The techniques that follow show how to use our thinking brain to our advantage.

## SHIFT YOUR PERSPECTIVE: COGNITIVE REAPPRAISAL

You've probably seen an image like this with a big cat like a lion or cheetah chasing a zebra or a gazelle. Both the animal chasing and the one being chased are in the middle of an acute physiological stress response and in a fight for their lives. Both animals have the physical stress attributes of increased heart rate, respiratory rate, and blood vessel constriction.

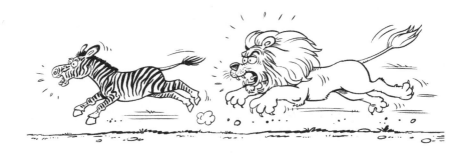

If the zebra gets caught, it will be eaten and die. If the lion fails to catch the zebra, it could starve and die. The difference between these two animals, the hunted and the hunter, is that the zebra is having what psychologists call a *threat* stress response and is experiencing fear. The lion is having a *challenge* stress response, experiencing excitement.

Both threat stress and challenge stress produce similar physical reactions, faster breathing, faster heartbeat, constricting blood vessels, all to help meet the threat or challenge effectively. In our bodies, the feelings of fear and the feelings of excitement are similar, but we experience the feelings of fear and excitement very differently, so catching ourselves when we are in a state of fear and using our brains to think our way into a state of excitement is a powerful, powerful skill.

Why? Because researchers have found that threat stress, over time, produces all the mental and physical problems we've discussed, but challenge stress does not. Additionally, a challenge stress response actually improves resilience and strengthens the immune system. In other words, we do well when we're excited with challenge stress but not when we're afraid and have threat stress.

In this section, we are going to look at the technique psychologists and neuroscientists call *cognitive reappraisal*, which is about how we can use our brains—in particular our prefrontal cortex—to shift our way of thinking about stress to turn fear stress into excitement or challenge stress. With cognitive reappraisal we use our thinking brain to reassess a situation, tell a different story about it, and feel inspired to rise to the challenge rather than get deflated.

There's fascinating research on this topic. In one study, done by Jeremy Jamieson, Matthew Nock, and Wendy Berry Mendes as a collaboration between Harvard University and UCSF, the scientists took a group of volunteers to test their response to what most people agree is highly stressful—public speaking.

The volunteers were randomly divided into three groups:

* *The first group was a control group, to which the researchers gave no instructions of any kind.*

* *The second group was told to ignore the stress when they experienced it.*

* *The third group was shown how to use cognitive reappraisal to reframe their thinking about public speaking.*

The researchers told the first group to give their presentation, told the second group to ignore their stress, and taught the third group how to shift their perspective and reappraise the situation. The researchers explained that the stress response has evolved to help us improve performance in stressful situations. By actively relabeling feelings of fear and turning them into an opportunity or challenge, the group was able to then reappraise the situation.

The researchers then went about measuring the stress responses of all volunteers in the three groups. They measured their stress responses in two ways: first, they measured total peripheral resistance, the amount of constriction in the blood vessels of the hands and feet, and second, the level of cardiac output as a measure of how hard the heart was pumping in liters per minute.

The reappraisal group had significantly better physiological responses than the control group or the group told to ignore the stress.

Normally when we experience an activating event, like being told we're going to give a speech, we have a physiologic arousal: our hearts beat faster, our palms sweat, and so on. Next, the brain tends to make a negative assessment about the situation, with a story such as, "Oh, I'm afraid I'm not going to do very well." "I'm going to bomb." "I hope my zipper isn't open." "I hate public speaking!"

When these kinds of negative stories or thoughts happen again and again, we become hypervigilant for threats, real and imagined. It's a case of the saying "what we practice will grow stronger." In addition, many of us come from cultures and backgrounds where being prepared for the worst, looking for the potential bad outcome, is our default way of looking at a situation. Others have bias toward negative appraisals or outcomes because of past painful or traumatic experiences.

If we don't consciously uproot these negative thought patterns, which often live under our conscious awareness, they can lead us to develop a habit of experiencing chronic threat stress similar to that of the zebra being chased by a lion *even when we aren't being threatened*.

With cognitive reappraisal, we still have the same initial physiological stress response, including increased heart rate, breathing rate, and blood vessel constriction, but we give ourselves the opportunity to reappraise or rethink our story. For example, you can say to yourself "I'm feeling afraid. This could be excitement. I can handle this situation." This kind of top-down reassessment calms your body and gives your mind a chance to intervene and redirect your thoughts."

Next, you can consciously call on your confidence and know-how to rise to the occasion. This act of conscious redirection shifts you from fear-mode to challenge-mode, enabling you to adapt or adjust your response.

Deciding to tell ourselves a story that can turn our fear into a challenge also breaks the pattern that triggers our unconscious search for threats during the process of giving a presentation. Also, this kind of conscious thinking can increase or enhance our performance. It is a very strong strategy for managing stress more effectively.

We can practice reappraisal by thinking about a situation that commonly causes us stress, like watching your child fall on the sports field or watching the stock market shrink our retirement savings. Notice the feeling of fear and then imagine what it would feel like to be challenged rather than frustrated or afraid. Really allow yourself to feel the call to action. Then think through how a determined person who is motivated to rise to the challenge would handle the situation. What steps are at your disposal? If the stock market is in free fall, how might you react to contain a panicky stress response? You could talk to an advisor. Or look at the long view of how the stock market goes up and down. You might even decide to sell. The point is this: you have choices.

The more you allow yourself to think through scenarios, the more control you assert over your own stress response. We can program ourselves to stop and redirect a cascade of negative thoughts and feelings. We can learn to shift from fear to challenge. And when we do this shift often enough, life is more fun and we not only feel better, we feel more in charge.

## CHOOSE TO ACT OR LET GO: THE CAN I/WILL I DECISION TREE

The "Can I change it or will I change it?" decision tree can help decrease worry, mental stuckness, and rumination (when your mind keeps spinning in circles) during times of prolonged crisis. Using this technique is very simple.

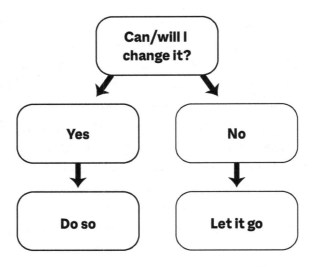

When you're focused on a particular situation that is bothering you, worrying you, or provoking anxiety, stop and ask yourself these questions:

1. *Is this something I can change?*

2. *If yes, ask yourself, "Is it something I'm willing to change?"*

3. *If you can change it and you're willing to do so, make the change.*

4. *If you can't change it or are unwilling to change it, can you let it go?*

A general rule of thumb is if a situation involves another person, system, or organization, it is less stressful to focus on what we ourselves can do as part of the dynamic, rather than on what we'd like other people to do or change. How can I change my own actions, thoughts, reactions, responses to make this situation better for myself? If there's something I can do, then I do it. If there isn't, then

I can give myself permission to stop stressing about it and focus my attention elsewhere.

For example, my nightly dose of 10 Oreo cookies is making me fat and that's stressing me out. I can change my snack from Oreos to an apple and that's a change I'm willing to make. On the other hand, my friend who is a popular gospel singer strongly believes that we are overreacting to the new coronavirus. I am not able to change her mind or get her to quit posting harmful things on social media. So what are my options? Either I can fixate on my friend's behavior and become more frustrated, or I can treat her point of view as a balloon on a string and let it go.

If the situation or concern is something we can change and are willing to change, by all means, we should go for it. This choice decreases the stress associated with a situation. If we cannot change it or we're not willing to change it, then we can make a conscious decision to let it go. And sometimes we will need to let go of stuff over and over again until we learn how not to stew on our negative thoughts.

When we get clear and keep our focus on things we can change, it decreases our stress overall. Taking the time to figure out what we are and aren't going to tackle right now can free up the time and energy we need to stay focused and healthy during this time. The serenity prayer captures the spirit of this technique. "God grant me the serenity to accept the things I cannot change, the courage to change the things I can, and the wisdom to know the difference." That about sums it up.

## FOCUS YOUR FLASHLIGHT

When we hear the phrase "tunnel vision" these days, it's usually being used as a criticism of somebody not being able to stand back and see the bigger picture. Physiologically, tunnel vision is a natural part of the stress response and is nature's way of keeping us alive.

Under threat from a saber-tooth tiger hiding in the bushes, our brains automatically narrow our focus so that we only think about how to stay alive when faced with a physical threat.

This kind of tunnel vision is part of our built-in survival instinct. If we're about to get eaten, we don't want our attention taken up with the sound of the babbling brook next to us, or the sight of butterflies fluttering around the flowers. We want to focus on tiger, tiger, tiger until we get the heck out of there. In fact, most of us do this when our visual cortex reduces peripheral vision so that we can literally narrow our focus.

It makes sense that we narrow our focus when we have to deal with a direct threat like a patient who is getting combative in the ambulance or emergency department. It's good to stay focused until the actual threat has been mitigated and is unable to harm you or anyone else.

The problem with our evolution is that this tunnel vision has not adapted to modern life. When it comes to all the stressors out there, not the tiger in the bushes, of course, but bills that are overdue, the grocery store being out of toilet paper, and the COVID-19 that can threaten our loved-ones, our mind can bounce from one stressful thing to another, jacking up our overall anxiety.

In our fast-paced modern lives, our tunnel vision stress response often gets activated by situations that are better addressed by our thinking brains than our reactive brains. Our tunnel vision response can also get triggered by an accumulation of stressors, any one of which might be manageable if addressed by the thinking brain on its own. Together, they make us feel more like we're being chased by a pack of hungry tigers that all need to be constantly watched, rather than thinking of them as simply a list of tasks to tackle.

Dan Siegel says we can use this "flashlight beam" of our mind to our advantage by consciously directing it at what's important at any given moment. If our mind seems stuck on something scary, we turn our power of attention and direct our flashlight beam to an action we can take right now to make the situation a little bit better.

For example, when a fellow grocery shopper pulled down his face mask to sneeze unencumbered into the open air rather than into his mask, my mind bounced from how inconsiderate he was, to the now contaminated organic honey crisp apples, to my son who asked me to bring him home honey crisps, to wondering how often people sneeze on produce when I'm not there to see it.

Then I took a breath and shifted the focus of my mental flashlight beam to moving away from the sneezy shopper and to the fact that I could get apples from another grocery store in town. If we shift our focus to something positive, safe, and action oriented, even for a little bit, it can decrease our stress response.

# *Manage Your Emotions*

Our thoughts are fueled by our emotions, which are part of an instinctive network of reactions based in the limbic system. In order to assert top-down control of our thoughts, we need to see our emotions more objectively. The techniques that follow will help you build emotional resilience, an important dimension to your stress management arsenal.

## NAME YOUR FEELINGS

My first marriage only lasted five months. I was in my twenties and getting married was clearly the wrong thing to do, but some good things came out of the experience, one being I discovered psychotherapy. My therapist at the time Jack and I did walking therapy where we would walk in a park and have our conversation as opposed to me lying on a couch and him sitting in a lounge chair smoking a pipe.

During one of our sessions, I related to Jack that my then-wife had stayed out the entire night the night before and had come home at 5:00 a.m. so she could say goodbye to me before I went to work.

Jack said, "Well, how did that make you feel?"

I responded by saying, "Well, it was the first time that she's done anything like this and blah, blah, blah."

"Okay, tell me how that made you feel."

I said, "Well, she was living with her parents when we met and she moved out and moved in with me. So this is her first real time out in the world and living on her own, and I don't blame her for wanting to sow her oats a little bit."

Jack grabbed my arm, spun me around, got right up in my face, and in a stern voice he said, "I asked you how that made you feel!"

And I said, "I guess I don't understand your question," which was a clue that I had a bit of a problem.

There's a psychological diagnosis called *alexithymia—a* for without, *lex* for words, *thymia* for emotion—for when people can't describe their emotions. At the time of this early marriage, I was a young paramedic. During paramedic school, I had learned all kinds of information about pharmaceuticals, and caring for people with diabetic emergencies, and gunshot wounds, and heart attacks; I'd learned how to read the EKGs, and the like.

However, without realizing it, I also learned to suppress my natural emotions. Most patients don't want a paramedic to be all emotional when they show up to the scene of their car accident. They want a paramedic who is cool, calm, and reassuring, and I was determined to be that kind of person. But what I hadn't realized was that distancing myself from my natural emotional reactions would become a hardened part of who I was.

So my therapy at the time became all about learning how to connect with my emotions. Since then, I have learned that having the ability to recognize and label my emotions in the moment is a powerful stress management tool—one that has made me more able to deal with tough situations and help others on their worst days. I've learned to label many different feelings. Before I would just say, "I'm mad." Now I can be more nuanced: Am I mad? Or perhaps annoyed? Disappointed? Frustrated? Irritated? Resentful? Afraid? Nervous? Uneasy? Worried?

You get the picture. The more we try to figure out how to label a feeling or emotion more specifically, the more we are able to deal with or manage the discomfort of that feeling.

The same goes for positive feelings. Give yourself some room to explore positive emotions, too. Are you happy? Grateful? Joyful? Relieved? Excited?

As human beings, we have an extensive array of possible emotions, and when we explore this vast range and learn to label them more precisely, we give ourselves a powerful stress-buster. It doesn't matter what the emotion is; the ability to label it helps decrease our stress response.

For some people, myself included, it really gives us more control over the feeling itself so that it doesn't get in our way when we are trying to be efficient on the front line or in a crisis. For many people, the first clue that they are having an emotion is noticing something physical. It is this physical feeling that works like a call to action to label the emotion. The earlier you notice the emotion and label it, the less likely it is to hijack your world.

For instance, am I clenching my fist? Has my heart rate increased? Am I raising my voice and snapping at people? Are my thoughts racing, or are my palms sweaty? Am I clenching my teeth? Am I acting controlling, being possessive, making threats, or just thinking negative thoughts? Am I feeling extra kind, or empathic, or vulnerable, or am I feeling like I am on the verge of tears, or that I just need to take a nap right now?

These physical signals are tied to specific emotions. The first step in learning how to name our emotions is becoming aware of them.

The more we can learn about identifying emotions and give them a label, the better able we will be to identify the trigger for that feeling. What caused me to clench my fist? Why is my heart racing? When you can trace the source of a feeling or reaction, you build your emotional resilience.

One of my favorite stories is about my son, Ax. At the time, he was eight years old and eating rigatoni with marinara sauce. He likes a lot of marinara sauce on his rigatoni, and he likes to eat in front of the television set, which I know is bad parenting, but Sascha and I let him do it a fair amount anyway. That evening, he still had about half a bowl left and he was carrying his bowl back into the kitchen when he tripped on one of his many Legos. He's got a lot of Legos. And I was watching Sascha, who was standing right there as this whole scene unfolded.

You've got to know one thing about Sascha: she really likes white things. We have white sofas, white club chairs, a white table, white paint on the walls. So this marinara was mid-flight, being spread as if it were a Jackson Pollock Rorschach-style red painting all over her white things.

As I watched, Sascha took a quick breath and actually said to herself under her breath, "What am I really feeling right now?"

And she said, "Surprise. I'm feeling surprised."

And then she looked at our son and said, "Ax, I'm feeling surprised. Are you feeling surprised?"

And he looked up and was like, "I'm surprised that 'surprise' is the word that's coming out of your mouth right now, Mom."

And she said, "Well, let's just clean this up."

And they just got together and cleaned it up.

Without the ability to catch and label an emotion in the moment, it would have been a very different scene—a pretty upset mom and a feeling bad little kid. Instead, it was just a parent and child working together to clean up a mess.

So, the next time something happens that makes you have a sudden strong feeling, stop for a moment and think: What am I really feeling right now? Even if what you're feeling in the moment really is anger or fear, by labeling the emotion, you activate that thinking brain and give yourself more choices about how to respond to the situation from a place of centeredness.

Check in with yourself right now. What emotion are you feeling? How were you feeling when you woke up today? Developing the emotional labeling habit will support you through all kinds of stressful situations at work and at home.

## SCHEDULE A WORRY SESSION: STIMULUS CONTROL TRAINING

Scheduling a time to worry likely seems counterintuitive to stress management. Many people think, *"Isn't stress management about not worrying or getting away from worry?"*

The thing is, some of us experience trying to *not* worry as another thing that turns up the volume on worry. Cognitive behavioral therapists suggest that instead of trying to avoid worrying, scheduling a worry session gives us the opportunity to ruminate for a while and then let it go. This strategy is known as *stimulus control training*.

The general practice is to allow for a 30-minute worry period. However, many of us might not have that much time these days. So whatever time is available—5 minutes, 10 minutes, or 20 minutes—anything up to but not beyond a half hour helps any kind of worries be brought to light, gives them a place to be worked out, and hopefully gives our minds a break. The recommendation is to schedule a once-daily worry session at least three hours before bedtime, regardless of when bedtime is. Why? Because a structured worrying period can sometimes interfere with sleep—and we already know that sleep is important to our overall health, well-being, resilience, and stress management.

During this scheduled worry time, try to worry as intensely as possible. Often when worries pop into our brain, we try to push them away or downplay them. During scheduled worry time, we really let it rip as intensely as possible, making sure to set a timer so we know when worry time is over.

And then, during the course of the day when worries pop up, we remind ourselves that we can postpone thinking about them until our next worry session. Some people like to keep a list of worries that pop up throughout the day so they can be sure to remember what they want or need to worry about, or so they can give a moment's acknowledgment to the worry without letting it take over non-worry time. Others might adopt the stance that if it's important enough, they will remember the worry and don't need to write it down. Whatever works, works.

When a worry session is over, move on to something else. Think of something else. Do something else. And don't replay or revisit the worry session. Let it go, knowing that tomorrow's worry session is another opportunity to dive in.

This strategy has been shown to be effective in reducing anxiety over time as well as in acute situations. There's something powerful about knowing that worry has a time and place where we can always come back to it but we don't need to carry it with us all day every day.

## EXPRESS GRATITUDE

Gratitude can be a powerful path for dialing down stress in the moment and on an ongoing basis. Studies have shown that cultivating gratitude results in improved emotional well-being. Two psychologists from University of California, Davis, Robert A. Emmons and Michael E. McCullough, describe gratitude as doing something for another person that results in a personal benefit that was not intentionally sought.

Why? Because whether it's thanking ourselves, another person, or mother nature, the action of expressing or feeling gratitude inspires happiness. It activates a parasympathetic nervous system response that enhances good mood, improves our sleep, improves our immune system, decreases pain, and can improve our interpersonal relationships.

There are a lot of ways to weave gratitude into our lives. Making a call to express gratitude or sending a text or e-mail to say thank you or give a compliment improves our own happiness and the happiness of the person who receives it. There's that old phrase that the scent of a rose lingers on the hand of the giver as well as the receiver. Expressing gratitude can be a way that we can manage stress for ourselves and for someone else. It has also been shown to improve work performance, especially in difficult situations. Gratitude also results in better group cohesiveness when it's expressed in a team environment.

The more we practice it, the more we feel it. Dan Siegel taught me that neurons that fire together wire together, meaning that the more we activate a particular neurologic pathway, the more likely it is for that pathway to be easily activated in the future. So, the more regularly we practice gratitude, the easier it is for us to feel grateful, regulate stress hormones in our body, decrease fear and anxiety, and build our emotional resilience. What a deal.

Some people use a gratitude journal as a way to write down the things they're grateful for. My wife, son, and I often practice doing a three-item gratitude list before going to sleep. Studies show that listing the things and people we're grateful for in the world just before we fall asleep actually enhances our ability to go to sleep.

Others ask themselves the question, What compliment would I like to give myself today? Self-gratitude is a powerful vehicle, and it's easy for people who are generally humble to forget that expressing self-gratitude is not only permissible but healthy.

Another strategy that helps is to have a gratitude buddy, someone they make an agreement with that they're going to share their gratitude with on a daily basis. Some people keep a gratitude jar at home. They write on little pieces of paper the things they're grateful for and add them to a clear, see-through jar. Whenever they're feeling a bit low, they can pull one or two out.

Since the pandemic started, I've been practicing conscious gratitude every time I wash my hands the requisite 20 seconds. It can be helpful to make a list of the people or animals in our lives that we're grateful for. My list includes nurses, physicians, physician's assistants, firefighters, paramedics, EMTs, police officers, hospital housekeeping staff, the mechanics that keep vehicles running, dispatchers in 911 call centers, farmers who grow the food I get to eat, the truckers who bring it to the grocery store, the grocery store workers who stock it on the shelves, the psychologists who are providing therapy to folks during this difficult time. Certainly, my wife and my son and the rest of our extended family are high on my list, as well as many more friends I know and friends I haven't met yet.

And you, my dear reader, I am deeply grateful for you and your willingness to take action to take care of yourself and decrease your own stress, which will have a positive impact on your life and those whose lives you touch.

## GROW YOUR AWARENESS:
## THE POWER OF MINDFULNESS

Developing a daily mindfulness practice is one of the most powerful ways to build and maintain resilience throughout the course of our lives. Years and years of studies support the benefits of meditation and mindfulness practice.

When meditation was first introduced into the United States, it was often thought of as some kind of hippy dippy Eastern practice.

But over time, and as more and more research has been done on its physical and emotional benefits, it has been embraced by all branches of the US Military.

One of my teachers, Richard Heckler, wrote a wonderful book called *In Search of the Warrior Spirit*, which talks about how meditative and contemplative practices have been practiced by the most elite units of the US Special Forces and have made them more effective at handling high stress situations. Now, all branches of the service have adopted meditation in various ways.

I've been fortunate in that I was introduced to meditation when I was 14 years old and have been meditating daily since then. I've explored a number of different styles of meditation and have found one that is centered around what Dan Siegel and his team at the Mindsight Institute in Los Angeles have created called the Wheel of Awareness. I blend it with influences from a few other disciplines. I've also read a number of wonderful books that have been published on the science behind and benefits of mindfulness meditation-type practices in the last few years.

A few years ago, I attended a lecture that Daniel Goleman gave on his book *Altered Traits*; I asked him: "So of all the different types of meditation that have been studied, which one do you think provides the most benefit?"

Without hesitation he said, "Whatever one you'll do. It's the actual doing of something that matters much more than any of the techniques that are involved."

Of the techniques that I have studied, including Vipassana meditation, Lomi-style mind-body meditation, transcendental meditation, and others, the Wheel of Awareness meditation is the most satisfying. Why? Because it feels like I'm taking my brain to the gym for a workout on attention and focus. I've been doing it daily for the last two years and I've upped my meditation practice to twice a day since COVID-19 hit.

Of all the meditation approaches and styles that I've tried, the Wheel of Awareness is the one with the most tangible, obvious benefits that happen for me instantly. All the credit for this goes to Dan Siegel. I highly encourage you to read his book *Aware*, which goes into exquisite depth on the subject of this practice. You can also find the link for his guided meditation on YouTube at the back of this book or if you Google the term *"Wheel of Awareness" meditation*.

❋ ❋ ❋

The basic concept of Siegel's practice is to use the image of a wheel with a hub at the center of it. The center or hub represents the experience of awareness itself. Around this hub, the spokes of the wheel are divided into four quadrants, representing different aspects of our human experience:

* *What we take in through our five senses*

* *The inner sensations of our body*

* *The activities of our mind*

* *The connection of our mind to things outside of us*

In the meditation, you move through the quadrants, focusing on each of the areas.

**FIRST QUADRANT** The first quadrant asks you to bring attention to your five senses, moving through each sense sequentially: first sight, then hearing, then taste, smell, and finally touch. I really enjoy using my sense of taste, and I especially like the taste of lemonade or dark chocolate melting in my mouth. Smell is the fourth one; it involves enjoying the olfactory sense, the smell of warm chocolate or freshly brewed coffee, or whatever scent comes to mind that is pleasing to you.

The fifth sense is the sense of touch. If I'm doing the meditation while sitting up or lying down or whatever, wherever I happen to be doing it, I just notice my clothes against my skin, or the sense of the pressure of my legs and my back against the chair that I'm in, and I just notice everything that's touching my skin.

**SECOND QUADRANT**   You then move on to the second quadrant of the wheel, which asks that you scan your body, releasing any tension or tightness in any area. I do this from my head to my feet just to keep it sequential. I start with my brain and the interior of my face and try to soften my facial muscles. I imagine relaxing my brain and making it soft. And then I do the same with my neck and down through my shoulders and arms, feeling my arms, kind of elongating and spreading out my attention throughout my body.

After the body scan, I spend a minute or two to simply enjoy my entire body being relaxed.

**THIRD QUADRANT**   The third quadrant is made up of mental activities, which include your emotions, thoughts, and beliefs. Now that your body is calm (or calmer), you turn to what's going on in your mind. For many of us, our minds are often full of chatter. At this point in the meditation, you are not trying to empty or erase the chatter or stream of thoughts and feelings; rather, Siegel suggests, you simply become aware of what the stream is—you observe thoughts, feelings, images.

He asks us to witness how our own thoughts arrive and leave our mind, to just notice as they come and go. Then, at this point, Siegel recommends bending the imaginary spoke of the wheel back into the center hub and enjoying the feeling of being aware of awareness itself. For me, this return feels much more like my traditional meditation, where I soften and allow things to go deep.

**FOURTH QUADRANT** After spending time and enjoying the depths of the hub, which for me feels very calm and centered, you can then proceed to the last quadrant of the wheel, which is all about relationships. Here, I imagine myself starting by putting my arms around my little family and feeling the warmth of that embrace, then I consciously expand this energy out to my community.

I think about putting my arms around everyone in my local and professional communities, both of which are wide and deep and scattered all over the world; I imagine gathering them into a large hug and drawing them close to me, imagining that the embrace includes everyone in Santa Barbara. I then take another breath and expand that out to the entire state of California. And then on the next breath, I embrace the entire country of the United States. Finally, I take a breath and really push it out to expand toward the entire planet and the entire world.

I sit with this connection and allow the energy of the embrace of the entire planet to sit with me. Sometimes, I transition that image into a loving kindness meditation where I say to myself, "May all beings be happy. May all beings be healthy. May all beings be free of suffering." And then I allow my eyes to drift open and I finish up. For me, this practice can take 5 minutes or up to 20 minutes, rarely much more.

Once you have a sense of how mindfulness feels, you can create small or brief opportunities during the course of the day to drop into mindfulness, even when it's a crazy, busy day. Dealing with danger, wearing personal protective equipment, the nonstop stress of people who need help, and caring for sick people can be overwhelming. With all that, it is very useful to have a mental practice that helps return us to a calm, mindful state of being.

Here's a mindfulness mini-exercise: When I take time to enjoy a cup of coffee or a cup of tea during the day, just for a few seconds or a minute I don't look at my phone or do anything except immerse myself in the warm cup. I smell the drink and let the aroma capture my full attention. When I take my first sip, I really taste it, let the flavor and warmth fill my mouth, allow myself to pause for a moment and be totally present with what I'm doing and where I'm at. Then I get back in action.

For me, another favorite way to do this mindfulness exercise is to use chocolate. In case you haven't noticed, I've mentioned chocolate a few times during the course of this book, and chocolate is a truly magical substance. Chocolate has one of the most complex smells on the planet and it contains phenylethylamine and tryptophan (the precursor for serotonin), which are believed to enhance mood and even have aphrodisiac effects.

So, when I unwrap a piece of chocolate, I just pause for a second and smell it and let the aromatherapy work. Then I take a small bite and let it sit in my mouth. A good quality chocolate will melt at a temperature that's just a bit lower than body temperature, so I can allow it to melt in my mouth rather than chewing. I let the flavors coat the tongue and the inside of the mouth and fully enjoy the experience for at least a moment before I wolf down the rest of it.

Remember, we can pause during the day for brief moments of extra mindfulness, knowing that it helps us manage our overall stress.

# WE ARE
# ALL IN THIS
# TOGETHER

# *Connect with Nature*

I grew up in Colorado where camping and hiking were a big part of my life. We now live in Santa Barbara, which is a blessing for which we are very grateful. One of the practices we have as a family is to get up together early in the morning before the sun rises, snuggle up on the sofa, and watch out the front window for the birds to wake up. My son calls it the bird show. There's something about just watching and connecting with the birds flying around in front of our home that is a really lovely start to the morning.

We don't have to live in a tropical oasis, seaside town, or the mountains to connect with nature. My wife Sascha's family lives in New York City, so we visit the great metropolis regularly. We always make time to hang out in Central Park during these visits. Playing on the rocks, in the playgrounds, walking, running, getting snacks from the vendors, and people-watching have been a reliable source of joy and happiness for our family.

Based on my observations of the people we interact with during our park outings, it seems to be a shared experience. Exposure to nature has well-documented benefits, including a better state of mind, a better state of emotional well-being, and physical health. Some interesting research has been done on this connection between nature and wellness. Mary Carol Hunter, Brenda Gillespie, and Sophie Yu-Pu Chen at the University of Michigan published a study in *Frontiers of Psychology* called "Urban Nature Experiences Reduce Stress in the Context of Daily Life Based on Salivary Bio-markers." These researchers took a group of volunteers in upstate Michigan and sampled their salivary cortisol and alpha amylase, hormones and enzymes that indicate stress, before and several times during their experiment. The volunteers were instructed to spend 10 minutes or more in an outdoor space that brought them in contact with nature.

Participants could choose where to go: some may have gone to a park for a walk or sat on their front step and gazed at a flower in a pot, whatever they chose. They could sit or walk. But no matter what they chose, doing it for 10 minutes or more, three times a week, dropped their cortisol rate by 23 percent and their alpha amylase rate by 28 percent. The biggest impact was for people who had a 20- to 30-minute contact with an outdoor space that gave a sense of nature.

Investing this amount of time connecting with nature has an immediate impact and offers you a huge boost in stress management. As with many of these techniques, some is better than none. Those of us who do not have much time still benefit from allowing ourselves even just a few minutes to connect with a flower or a tree in the world around us. Making a point of noticing nature connection opportunities in our day-to-day lives can help us build resilience, help us reduce our stress levels, make us feel better, and arm us with a powerful technique to manage stress more effectively.

# *Make Connection Happen*

L oneliness is a bigger risk factor for early death than obesity or smoking. Loneliness is the feeling of isolation. The solitude associated with physical distancing can exacerbate feelings of loneliness. It's possible to feel lonely and disconnected when surrounded by people.

Much of the research around addressing loneliness focuses on what are called *social facilitation interventions*. These involve activities with groups of people. Although these activities are less available during a pandemic, many other online gatherings are happening around all kinds of topics. From house concerts to 12-step meetings, to virtual happy hours, yoga classes, dance parties, and dog and cat owner meetups, there is likely something for everyone. A quick search came up with online gatherings for introverts, atheists, corrections officers, critical care nurses, EMTs, and transgender stay-at-home moms.

In a recent lecture I attended, psychiatrist and neuroscience researcher Bruce Perry noted that before we are born, we do not experience hunger or thirst. We are surrounded by warm fluid, soothed by the constant sound and vibrations from our mother's body and heartbeat. This is really our first relationship, our first connection.

One strategy that can help re-create this feeling of our first connection is to climb into a warm bath, dim the lights, and listen to a playlist of songs with 60–80 beats per minute (bpm), the same rhythm as our mother's heartbeat. Some of my favorites are "Bridge Over Troubled Water" by Simon and Garfunkel (79 bpm), "Dream On" by Aerosmith (80 bpm), "Susie" by the Rolling Stones (80 bpm), "Every Rose Has Its Thorn" by Poison (70 bpm), "Desperado" by the Eagles (60 bpm), "I Guess That's Why They Call It the Blues" by Elton John (60 bpm), "Stagger Lee" by the Grateful Dead (74 bpm), and "Fire on the Mountain" also by the the Grateful Dead (76 bpm). You can also find a few websites that list the beats per minute of all kinds of songs to help you build a personal playlist that suits your taste in music.

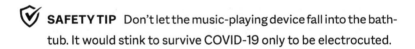 **SAFETY TIP** Don't let the music-playing device fall into the bathtub. It would stink to survive COVID-19 only to be electrocuted.

For those of us who live alone during this time of physical distancing, it can be difficult to get the relaxation and comfort that comes from an actual human hug. Pets can help fill this void. Our cat, Cleo, really seems to be enjoying having us at home all of the time and we enjoy her company just as much. It can help to take time to give yourself a foot massage, a hand massage, or a shoulder rub, it can also help to serve yourself a proper meal at the table, take yourself on a stay-at-home date, and give yourself credit for treating yourself well. Treating yourself well is an important part of keeping yourself in shape to help others.

One other strategy to combat loneliness is to reach out and connect on the phone or via video chat with someone else who might be feeling lonely. If they are feeling bad, reaching out can really help them, whether it's a quick touching-base check-in or a longer visit. My wife has made an internal commitment to call her mother, who we're physically distancing from, every morning and evening. These calls sometimes last less than a minute, but it's good for both of them to know that they are there for each other. When it comes to loneliness it's really hard to help someone else without helping ourselves, too.

# Stay Open: The Importance of Family and Friends

M y sister Sue Taigman taught me something that she and her colleague Craig Ross from the international consulting firm Verus Global call the *Homeward Bound Framework*. The principle of the framework is based on the observation that with taxing jobs, we often come home exhausted, and our families, the people who mean more to us than anyone else, get the dregs of our energy.

The goal is to save some of the best you have to offer for the people at home. These questions are designed for you to ask yourself before you walk in the door and connect with your family:

1. *What did I learn today that is valuable?*

2. *What did I do well today?*

**3.** *What are the three greatest blessings in my life?*

**4.** *How can I be the best [mom, dad, spouse, friend] I've ever been when I walk in the door?*

During non-pandemic times, I travel roughly 41 weeks a year for work. I was always happy to see my wife and son when I got home, but it seemed like we'd often end up in an argument within a few minutes or hours of me walking in the door.

I'd been giving my best to clients, partners, students, and colleagues while getting lousy sleep in hotels and eating travel food. Although I was thrilled to be home, I was not bringing home my best.

I started using the Homeward Bound Framework four or five years ago after learning it from my wise and wonderful sister. As I was writing this section of the book, my wife said, "I didn't know you were doing that. It really works; we haven't had any of those daddy's home arguments in years."

Whether intentional or not, most of us have our own homecoming ritual, and it's likely that the pandemic has caused it to change. It's helpful to ask our families what they need when we come home and what they need when we go off to work in a world with new dangers. We should assume we don't really know what they need or want from us unless we have that conversation with them. Having a real discussion about these frequent transition points can enrich our relationships and decrease everyone's stress.

I encourage you to share the techniques in this book with your family, however you define family. Chances are very good that they are feeling anxious too. If the folks in our circle each have a preferred stress management technique, we can be more helpful when we notice stress taking its toll on them. Reminding someone to wiggle their toes, take a few tactical breaths, or find the excitement in their fear is more effective if they've learned about it beforehand.

**SAFETY TIP** Get permission to offer your loved ones stress management techniques before offering them. "Would you like a stress management technique right now?" gives the other person the chance to say, "No! Just hug me!"

When it comes to sharing stress management techniques with family or friends, we suggest that you try one or two together. Then, as a family, pick one and say, "OK, for today, we're going to do tactical breathing when we feel stressed, and we're going to practice it together at the beginning of the day." And then encourage everyone to try it throughout the day.

Then, when you come back together at the end of the day, each person can take a turn talking about how it worked for them and what they learned so that everyone can support each other in the practice and process. If we can let our stress management team members and family members feel like equals in the process, it works better than if we try to make ourselves into the teachers and them into students. Maintaining a spirit of curiosity and fun, especially with kids, is important to keeping everyone in it together.

During times when we are under severe stress, as we are now in the COVID-19 crisis, it's important to stay open in our communications, particularly with our kids. Kids can figure out when we're stressed, and they take their cues about how worried to be from their parents and other adults in their lives.

If they ask about COVID-19, tell them just enough. Make it age-appropriate, with just enough information for them to feel they're getting the truth. If they think that we're hiding something, they simply get scared and their imaginations run wild. On the other hand, too much information can cause unnecessary fear. We know our kids, we know our families. We can trust our instincts on how much—and what—to share.

My experience is that kids tend to ask questions like these:

*What is coronavirus?*

*How do you get it?*

*Will I die if I get it?*

*Will you die if you get it?*

Answering their questions simply and honestly is important. Limiting their exposure to the news and keeping our eyes open for unusual ways that kids might ask for reassurance is also important. We might be asked to play and build Legos more frequently. They might ask more questions than usual or require more attention. *Where does that bird live? Why is the cream cheese so thick on my bagel? When will I be able to play with my friends?* And that's just the tip of the iceberg.

These are requests for reassurance. The act of responding and taking our kids' questions seriously lets them know we are there for them.

*I'm not sure where the bird lives. Where do you think it lives?*

*Do you like the cream cheese thick or do you prefer it a different way?*

*You'll be able to play with your friends when it is safe to do so. My number one job is to help keep you healthy and safe, so for now, we can do video play dates, and when it is safe, we'll get back together in real life. I'm glad we get to be together now.*

Keeping communication channels open and using this together-time to stay connected in loving, kind ways can help the entire family dial down the stress as a team.

Your family might also want to try meditating together. Turning on one of our phones with one of Dan Siegel's Wheel of Awareness guided meditations is a pretty regular practice in our house and one that we all enjoy. It's also fascinating to watch our eight-year-old really get into a deeply meditative state.

And don't forget that the kids really pick up on conversations we have with other folks. They tend to hear and understand way more than we might give them credit for. So just be aware of their minds at work and play as you communicate with them.

# *Be a Leader*

E veryone on the front line exercises leadership in their day-to-day interactions with the public. For that reason, we all have an extra responsibility when it comes to managing our own stress response and helping those around us manage stress as well. As leaders, we have the power to create a collective stress management solution.

How does this work?

The limbic system that controls our emotions is an *open loop system*, which means that individuals affect others with whom they are in contact. In other words, each of us has the ability to positively affect other people's stress hormone levels, cardiovascular functions, sleep rhythms, and immune functions.

You can see this phenomenon when you're in a group of people and one person yawns, and then that yawn becomes contagious. This is a manifestation of the open loop nature of the limbic system. We've also seen that when we calm down and exhibit signs of calmness, others can respond by calming down. Regular breathing, centered movements, relaxed facial expressions, and eye contact all signal an internal state of centeredness that helps those around us find a more calm, grounded place inside.

As a leader—whether you have a formal title or not—keep in mind that people take their cues from you. It's like having a bunch of people riding behind you on the roller coaster. Your emotions are out in front, in the first car. If your emotions are going up and down and topsy-turvy and sideways, your entire team is affected. We have the power to lead with positive thoughts and channeled emotions.

This brings to mind one of my earliest experiences of good leadership in crisis circumstances. One of my early bosses as a paramedic was Norm Dinerman, a physician who was the director of the Denver Paramedic Division and also worked as an attending physician in the emergency department at Denver General Hospital.

Denver General was a Level 1 Trauma Center and it had residents and interns and medical school students and nursing students and paramedic students—it was the place that received all the worst of the major traumas in the City and County of Denver. People who worked there affectionately called the emergency department the "DG Knife and Gun Club."

It was often very hectic. As paramedics, we'd bring in a patient with a gunshot or a stab wound, and we'd see 25 or 30 people in the trauma room. We'd hear lots of noise and feel the chaos as people descended on the patient to take care of them—except for when Norm Dinerman was the attending physician.

When Norm was on duty, the same 25 or 30 people were there, but the emergency department would be absolutely pin-drop silent. Norm would calmly say to me as the young paramedic coming in, "Mike, what do you have for us?" And I would give my report about the nature of the patient. I was always able to deliver that report faster and more succinctly when Norm was there because I wasn't being interrupted and didn't have to repeat anything. I'd give the report as we moved the patient over to the main trauma bed.

And then Norm would say, "Does anyone have any questions for the paramedic?" "No?" "Thank you, Mike." And then he would very clearly choreograph all the other movements of critical patient intervention and trauma care.

Some friends of mine decided to time the trauma room treatment from when a patient arrived to when they went to the operating room. They discovered that patients actually got faster care when Norm was on as an attending, even though it felt like everything was happening more slowly because it was so quiet, so choreographed, and so precise. The calm, deliberate, orderly feeling Norm established allowed everybody to relax and do their best work caring for critical patients.

I have tried to emulate Norm's sense of calm throughout my life in my own leadership positions.

So, how can we promote a calm, effective work environment for our teams?

First, we need to make sure we connect with our people at a deep level. Although we may have been trained to think it's inappropriate to ask people how they're feeling or how they're doing, in times of prolonged crisis like this, those guidelines need to go out the window.

It is incredibly important to make real connections with the people we work with. Ask them how they're doing and when they say, "fine," know that *fine* may stand for fouled up, insecure, needy, and emotional.

So, when we ask our teammate that question again, "No, how are you really doing? How's your family doing?" take the time to connect and listen to their response. Make it more than a check-the-box conversation. Make it a real connection.

Investing the energy to connect during downtime can help make us work more efficiently when it's time to act. This approach also helps keep the whole team's stress levels down so they can feel more confident, calm, and effective at work and at home. Asking questions and listening to people shows leadership and helps our teammates dial-down their own stress.

Here is another tip: we need to make sure our people have the time they need to maintain personal protective equipment (PPE) requirements and take care of basic bodily needs like eating, drinking, and relieving themselves. When we're working in a healthcare setting where we are in PPE throughout the course of our shift, it takes time and skill to remove that equipment to eat safely without contaminating the food and contaminating ourselves.

Being in charge means that we need to build time into the schedule structures for our teams to be able to eat, to hydrate, to go to the bathroom. These are all basic life functions that can get impaired when you're working in a crisis-oriented healthcare situation with a contagious pathogen in the environment, reinforcing the need for you and your team to wear PPE.

Those of us who aren't in charge need to let superiors know what's not working with new protocols so that adjustments can be made. A little lapse can mean somebody contracts a disease that may cause them to lose their life or they may bring it home to somebody in their family.

As leaders, it's our job to support, nurture, and keep everyone safe, regardless of our place in the organizational hierarchy.

# *Personalize Your Stress Management Toolbox*

R eading this book is a great first step toward building an approach and a set of go-to tools that help you super-charge your stress management during times of extraordinary stress. The next step is to try to practice some of these tools in your daily life so that you learn what works for you and what doesn't. There is no one-size-fits-all.

How do we do that? Here, I share a simplified version of a system that's been used all over the world to make dramatic improvements. In the healthcare world, there is a big gap between when a new treatment has been proven through scientific research to be beneficial to patients and when the majority of people who need it get the benefit of the new treatment. One study published in the *Journal of the Royal Society of Medicine* showed a 17-year gap between knowing what helps patients and patients getting the treatment. One of the systems used to help close that gap and make all kinds of other improvements in healthcare is *improvement science*. Improvement science is the science of making changes that work, bringing knowledge into action in real life.

One of the most powerful and popular tools in improvement science is the Model for Improvement created by the Austin, Texas-based Associates in Process Improvement. Here is the model:

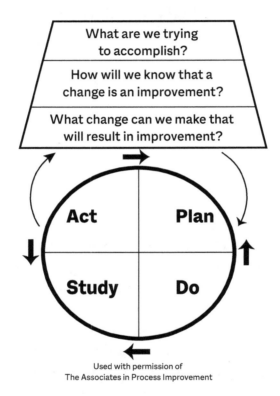

Used with permission of
The Associates in Process Improvement

The first part of this model sets us up for a clear goal and a clear way of knowing whether what we're doing is working. For our purposes, the answer to the first question, "What are we trying to accomplish?" is reduce threat stress, improve resilience, and improve happiness for ourselves. If this answer does not ring true for you, then make up your own. It could be to improve sleep, feel less trashed at the end of a work shift, bring the best you home from work, or whatever else matters most to you.

The next question, "How will we know that change is an improvement?" focuses on what you can measure to know that you're making progress. This is a personal feedback system that lets you know if the stress management technique you're using is helping you or not.

For example, I've been focusing on improving my sleep, so I track the number of hours of sleep and the number of minutes of deep sleep I get each night. Some people track how frequently they feel an internal sense of panic; others notice how stressed they feel on a scale of 1 to 10 just before connecting with their family. Sascha tracks the intensity of happiness she and our son experience when she gives him a big hug first thing in the morning when she sees him after he wakes up. I encourage you to track something that's easy, meaningful, and aligned with your desired accomplishment.

Next, ask yourself, "What change can I make that will result in improvement?" This is where you get to choose one or more of the techniques in this book. And remember, the best one is the one you use. We are all different, so there's no right or wrong answer to which technique to try first.

The second part of the model, Plan, Do, Study, Act (PDSA), is where you get to take action and do what's called *small tests of change*. I've simplified this part of the model for our purposes here. Essentially, this is your try-it, test-it, keep-it, or trash-it phase.

**FIRST, DECIDE WHAT TO TRY AS A TECHNIQUE AND WHEN TO TRY IT.** And right now is just fine. The key to making this step valuable is to make a prediction of what you think is going to happen when you try a technique. For example, if you want to try the pulling-the-carpet-back-with-your-toes technique from GRACE, predict how it will feel.

**NEXT, GIVE IT A TRY.** Notice how natural or unnatural pulling your toes back feels. Was it easy to do? Hard? Keep track of how you feel and any thoughts or judgements you have as you try toe-wiggling, breathing, imagining a pleasant smell or taste, or any of the other techniques.

**NEXT, STUDY.** Don't overthink this step. It's all about doing a quick comparison between your initial prediction and what your real results were. Did you think pulling your toes back would feel weird? In actuality, was it kind of interesting? Again, you are not judging your reactions; you are observing them.

**NEXT, ACT.** Here's when you ask yourself if the technique or strategy worked for you. If it worked, then you'll want to keep it, meaning keep using it and get it ingrained in your implicit memory. You notice you're becoming stressed, you go to this technique to stay centered. If it worked OK, but you also thought of a way to adapt it a bit, you might want to make that adjustment. For example, modifications that enhance the effectiveness for you could be adding ankle rolls to the wiggling-toe technique, making noise on the exhale with deep breathing, or tapping your temples or collar bones to mimic the rhythm of a heartbeat during sensory awareness practice.

And of course, if the technique just didn't work for you at all, then you can trash it—abandon it and choose another one to try.

The main benefit of using this improvement science–based approach is that it helps interesting ideas become real skills that provide real help. Once you get the hang of it, you can use this proven framework to improve anything in your personal or professional life.

# *We Can Do It*

T he techniques offered in this book are not designed to take our stress levels from super-high to zero. That really is not possible and isn't the intent of the book. But they can take us from a high stress state to a moderate stress state and give us go-to strategies that work for us in the moment. With practice, these tools can help reduce the intensity, frequency, and duration of high threat stress moments so we can work better and lead better lives.

We hope you reach out to us online to share your thoughts and experiences. We also hope that you feel inspired to share what works for you with your colleagues and friends who are dealing with the same kinds of stuff. We each have the ability to support one another as we keep learning how to manage—or super-charge—our stress responses. As helpers, it's important to also allow ourselves to be helped by others as we get through the COVID-19 pandemic together.

# Resources

The company I work for offers a neuroscience-based training program called *ResilientFirst*. It's an app-based system built in collaboration with our Australian partners Hello Driven. It starts with a brief, scientifically validated, 16-question resilience assessment called the PR6. Then it drops you into a customized training program that takes less than 5 minutes a day to build your resilience. Check it out at *https://www.firstwatch.net/resilientfirst/*.

You may also want to check out Dan Siegel's Wheel of Awareness meditation: *https://www.youtube.com/watch?v=ODlFhOKahmk*.

Here are some books that you might find helpful if you're looking to deepen your knowledge on stress management and resilience:

*Executive Resilience: Neuroscience for the Business of Disruption* by Jurie Rossouw and Pieter Rossouw

*Aware: The Science and Practice of Presence—A Complete Guide to the Groundbreaking Wheel of Awareness Meditation Practice* by Daniel Siegel, M.D.

*Altered Traits: Science Reveals How Meditation Changes Your Mind, Brain, and Body* by Daniel Goleman and Richard Davidson

*Peace Is Every Step: The Path of Mindfulness in Every Day Life* by Thich Nhat Hanh

*In Search of the Warrior Spirit, Fourth Edition: Teaching Awareness Disciplines to the Green Berets* by Richard Strozzi-Heckler

*Tiny Habits: The Small Changes That Change Everything* by B.J. Fogg

*Why Zebras Don't Get Ulcers: The Acclaimed Guide to Stress, Stress-Related Diseases, and Coping* by Robert M. Sapolsky

*The Empathy Effect: Seven Neuroscience-Based Keys for Transforming the Way We Live, Love, Work and Connect Across Differences* by Helen Riess, Liz Neporent

*The Telomere Effect: A Revolutionary Approach to Living Younger, Healthier, Longer* by Elizabeth Blackburn and Elissa Epel

*UnDo It!: How Simple Lifestyle Changes Can Reverse Most Chronic Diseases* by Dean Ornish and Anne Ornish

*How Not to Die: Discover the Foods Scientifically Proven to Prevent and Reverse Disease* by Michael Greger

# References

## FIRST CALM YOUR BODY

Bersani, F. S., et al. (2016). Association of dimensional psychological health measures with telomere length in male war veterans. *Journal of Affective Disorders, 190*, 537-542. *https://doi.org/10.1016/j.jad.2015.10.037*

Blackburn, E., & Epel, E. (2017). *The telomere effect*. New York: Grand Central Publishing.

Castro, C. A., et al. (2006). Battlemind training: Building soldier resiliency. In *Human Dimensions in Military Operations-Military Leaders' Strategies for Addressing Stress and Psychological Support* (42-1-42-6). Meeting Proceedings RTO-MP-HFM-134, Paper 42.

Chen, S. H., Epel, E. S., Mellon, S. H., Lin, J., Reus, V. I., Rosser, R., Kupferman, E., Burke, H., Mahan, L., Blackburn, E. H., & Wolkowitz, O. M. (2014). Adverse childhood experiences and leukocyte telomere maintenance in depressed and healthy adults. *Journal of Affective Disorders, 169*, 86-90. *https://doi.org/10.1016/j.jad.2014.07.035*

Conklin, Q. A., et al. (2018). Insight meditation and telomere biology: The effects of intensive retreat and the moderating role of personality. *Brain, Behavior, and Immunity, 70*, 233-245. *https://doi.org/10.1016/j.bbi.2018.03.003*

De Baca, T. C., et al. (2017). Sexual intimacy in couples is associated with longer telomere length. *Psychoneuroendocrinology, 81*, 46–51. *https:// doi.org/10.1016/j.psyneuen.2017.03.022*

Elon Poll—COVID-19 Outbreak. (n.d.). Elon University. Retrieved April 12, 2020, from *https://www.elon.edu/u/elon-poll/elon-poll-COVID-19 -outbreak/*

Epel, E. S., et al. (2004). Accelerated telomere shortening in response to life stress. *Proceedings of the National Academy of Sciences, 101*(49), 17312–17315. *https://doi.org/10.1073/pnas.0407162101*

Epel, E. S., & Prather, A. A. (2018). Stress, telomeres, and psychopathology: Toward a deeper understanding of a triad of early aging. *Annual Review of Clinical Psychology, 14*, 371–397. *https://doi.org/10.1146 /annurev-clinpsy-032816-045054*

Fossel, M. (1997). *Reversing human aging.* Fort Mill, SC.

Goleman, D. (1995). *Emotional intelligence.* New York: Bantam.

Goglin, S. E., et al. (2016). Change in leukocyte telomere length predicts mortality in patients with stable coronary heart disease from the heart and soul study. *PLoS ONE, 11*(10). *https://doi.org/10.1371/journal .pone.0160748*

Greger, M. (2019). *How not to diet: The groundbreaking science of healthy, permanent weight loss.* Flatiron Books.

Greger, M., & Stone, G. (2015). *How not to die: Discover the foods scientifically proven to prevent and reverse disease.* Flatiron Books.

Kim, P. Y., Kok, B. C., & Thomas, L. J. L. (2012). *Land combat study of an army infantry division 2003–2009.* Silver Spring, MD: Walter Reed, 22.

Lai, J., et al. (2020). Factors associated with mental health outcomes among health care workers exposed to coronavirus disease 2020. *JAMA Network Open, 3*(3), e203976–e203976. *https://doi.org/10.1001 /jamanetworkopen.2020.3976*

MacKinnon, J. B. (2016, August 11). The strange brain of the world's greatest solo climber. *Nautilus. http://nautil.us/issue/39/sport/the-strange -brain-of-the-worlds-greatest-solo-climber*

Neria, Y., DiGrande, L., & Adams, B. G. (2011). Posttraumatic stress disorder following the September 11, 2001, terrorist attacks. *The American Psychologist, 66*(6), 429-446. *https://doi.org/10.1037/a0024791*

Ornish, D., & Ornish, A. (2019). *UnDo it!: How simple lifestyle changes can reverse most chronic diseases.* Ballantine Books.

Patterson, P. D., et al. (2012). Association between poor sleep, fatigue, and safety outcomes in Emergency Medical Services providers. *Prehospital Emergency Care: Official Journal of the National Association of EMS Physicians and the National Association of State EMS Directors, 16*(1), 86-97. *https://doi.org/10.3109/10903127.2011.616261*

Roediger, H. L. (1990). Implicit memory: Retention without remembering. Arlington, VA: *American Psychologist, 45,* 1043.

## USE YOUR BREATH: TACTICAL BREATHING

Grossman, D., & Christensen, L. (2008). *On combat, the psychology and physiology of deadly conflict in war and in peace* (3rd ed.). Warrior Science Publications.

## USE THE POWER OF YOUR BRAIN

Harvey, A., Nathens, A. B., Bandiera, G., & LeBlanc, V. R. (2010). Threat and challenge: Cognitive appraisal and stress responses in simulated trauma resuscitations. *Medical Education, 44*(6), 587-594. *https://doi.org/10.1111/j.1365-2923.2010.03634.x*

Jamieson, J. P., Nock, M. K., & Mendes, W. B. (2012). Mind over matter: Reappraising arousal improves cardiovascular and cognitive responses to stress. *Journal of Experimental Psychology. General, 141*(3), 417-422. *https://doi.org/10.1037/a0025719*

Seery, M. D. (2011). Challenge or threat? Cardiovascular indexes of resilience and vulnerability to potential stress in humans. *Neuroscience & Biobehavioral Reviews, 35*(7), 1603-1610. *https://doi.org/10.1016/j.neubiorev.2011.03.003*

## MANAGE YOUR EMOTIONS

Sancar, B., & Aktas, D. (2019). The relationship between levels of Alexithymia and communication skills of nursing students. *Pakistan Journal of Medical Sciences, 35*(2), 489–494. *https://doi.org/10.12669/pjms.35.2.604*

## SCHEDULE A WORRY SESSION

Borkovec, T. D., et al. (1983). Stimulus control applications to the treatment of worry. *Behavior Research and Therapy, 21*(3), 247–251. *https://doi.org/10.1016/0005-7967(83)90206-1*

## EXPRESS GRATITUDE

Emmons, R. A., & McCullough, M. E. (2003). Counting blessings versus burdens: An experimental investigation of gratitude and subjective well-being in daily life. *Journal of Personality and Social Psychology, 84*(2), 377–389. *https://doi.org/10.1037/0022-3514.84.2.377*

## GROW YOUR AWARENESS

Siegel, D. (2018). *Aware: The science and practice of presence—The groundbreaking meditation practice.* New York: Tarcher Perigee.

Strozzi-Heckler, R. (2007). *In search of the warrior spirit: Teaching awareness disciplines to the green berets* (4th ed.). Berkeley, CA: Blue Snake Books.

## CONNECT WITH NATURE

Hunter, M. R., Gillespie, B. W., & Chen, S. Y.-P. (2019). Urban nature experiences reduce stress in the context of daily life based on salivary biomarkers. *Frontiers in Psychology, 10. https://doi.org/10.3389/fpsyg.2019.00722*

## MAKE CONNECTION HAPPEN

Holt-Lunstad, J., Smith, T. B., Baker, M., Harris, T., & Stephenson, D. (2015). Loneliness and social isolation as risk factors for mortality:

A meta-analytic review. *Perspectives on Psychological Science.*
Retrieved April 19, 2020, from *https://journals-sagepub-com.ucsf*
*.idm.oclc.org/doi/full/10.1177/1745691614568352*

## STAY OPEN: THE IMPORTANCE OF FAMILY AND FRIENDS

Ross, C. W. (2012, September 24). Homeward bound. Verus Global. *https://*
*www.verusglobal.com/homeward-bound/*

## BE A LEADER

Goleman. (2014, February 9). Daniel Goleman: Understanding the science
of moods at work. *http://www.danielgoleman.info/daniel-goleman*
*-understanding-the-science-of-moods-at-work/*

Morris, Z. S., Wooding, S., & Grant, J. (2011). The answer is 17 years, what is
the question: Understanding time lags in translational research. *Jour-*
*nal of the Royal Society of Medicine, 104*(12), 510–520. *https://doi.org*
*/10.1258/jrsm.2011.110180*

## BUILDING A PERSONAL STRESS MANAGEMENT SYSTEM THAT WORKS FOR YOU

API—Associates in Process Improvement—Developing methods. (n.d.).
Retrieved April 25, 2020, from *http://www.apiweb.org/index.php*
*/services/developing-methods*

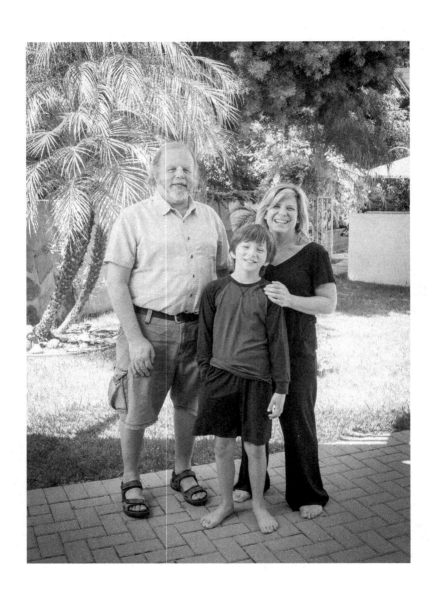

# *About the Authors*

## Mike Taigman

For several decades as a popular educator and author, Mike has focused on helping emergency medical services, fire, nurses, police, physicians, and other healthcare professionals take better care of themselves so they can take better care of their patients and communities.

Mike has authored more than 600 articles in professional journals and has worked with emergency services and healthcare organizations in 48 of the 50 states, most of the Canadian provinces, Israel, Palestine, Australia, and throughout Europe. His expertise includes stress management, resilience, EMS street survival, patient-centered leadership, and effective quality and performance improvement.

Mike worked as a Denver General street paramedic for over a decade, became a flight paramedic, and also served on the leadership team of several EMS organizations. Mike helped build some of the most innovative, most complex, and largest emergency medical systems in the nation.

Currently, Mike leads ResilientFirst, the neuroscience-based resilience training program offered by FirstWatch, and teaches improvement science at University of California, San Francisco's Master of Science in Healthcare Administration and Interprofessional Leadership program and at University of Maryland, Baltimore County's Master of Art in Emergency Health Services Management program. He also frequently serves as faculty for the Institute for Healthcare Improvement. He holds an MA in Organizational Systems.

For Mike, taking care of frontline personnel is the right thing to do on every level. This book is his offering to help his community get through the pandemic.

## Sascha Liebowitz

Sascha is a writer and author of *www.livingeveryminuteofit.com*, a blog about living each day with patience, tolerance, kindness, and love toward oneself and others. A former New York lawyer, she now lives in California and focuses on family, writing, and being of service to others. She holds a BA from Columbia College and a JD from New York University School of Law.

CPSIA information can be obtained
at www.ICGtesting.com
Printed in the USA
LVHW051419050720
659740LV00004B/312